SYNDROME X,
the Silent Killer

The New Heart Disease Risk

Gerald Reaven, M.D.

Terry Kristen Strom, M.B.A.

Barry Fox, PH.D.

A Fireside Book
Published by Simon & Schuster
New York London Toronto Sydney

FIRESIDE
Rockefeller Center
1230 Avenue of the Americas
New York, NY 10020

First Fireside Edition 2001
FIRESIDE and colophon are registered trademarks
of Simon & Schuster, Inc.
Designed by Meryl Sussman Levavi/Digitext, Inc.
Manufactured in the United States of America

10   9   8   7   6   5   4

The Library of Congress has cataloged the Simon & Schuster edition as follows:

Reaven, Gerald M.
    Syndrome X : overcoming the silent killer that can give you a heart attack /
Gerald Reaven, Terry Kristen Strom, Barry Fox.
        p.   cm.
    Includes bibliographical references and index.
        1. Coronary heart disease—Etiology.   2. Insulin resistence—Complications.
3. Coronary heart disease—Prevention.   4. Coronary heart disease—Diet therapy.
I. Strom, Terry Kristen.   II. Fox, Barry.   III. Title.
RC685.C6 R38 2000
616.1'23—dc21   99-052592
ISBN 0-684-86862-8
        0-684-86863-6 (Pbk)
Previoulsy published in hardcover as Syndrome X: Overcoming the Silent Killer That
Can Give You a Heart Attack.

NOTE TO READERS

ACKNOWLEDGMENTS

I am deeply indebted to all those medical researchers whose published results helped me form the scientific basis of my work and this book. In addition, I gratefully acknowledge the enormous contributions made by the medical students, research fellows and faculty colleagues I have had the privilege of collaborating with over the past forty years at Stanford University School of Medicine. It would be disingenuous of me to suggest that I did not play an important role in our joint efforts, but no medical investigator accomplishes anything without the help of many others. I have been exceptionally lucky, having so many truly talented and creative individuals on my research team. Without their help, this book would not have been possible.

Gerald Reaven, M.D.

A Note on Style

Although this book is the result of a close collaboration between the three authors, for the sake of convenience and clarity we have used the "I" voice of Gerald Reaven throughout. And when you see "we," that's Dr. Reaven speaking of his research group at Stanford University.

To all those researchers whose published results
have helped me form the scientific basis of my work
and this book.

CONTENTS

SYNDROME X,
the Silent Killer

The New Heart Disease Risk

A Little-Known

Problem

THE "UNKNOWN"

HEART SLAYER

BOB'S LIFE BEGAN TO unravel one night after he and his wife, Eleanor, finished a healthy, home-cooked dinner consisting of fresh sea bass, spinach salad, baked potato and asparagus tips, topped off with low-fat carrot cake to celebrate Bob's fifty-eighth birthday. Fish, vegetables and low-fat dressing on the salad: just the low-fat diet the doctor recommended.

Later that evening Bob took the couple's terrier, Cargo, out for an evening stroll. The birthday boy was looking forward to breathing in the crisp San Francisco air, but he also felt a little tired. And as he and Cargo headed toward the park he began to feel a slight pressure in his chest, right beneath his breastbone. Thinking it might be indigestion, Bob forced a burp to relieve the discomfort.

Later, at the park, Bob was still aware of the uncomfortable heaviness in his chest. He had suffered from indigestion before, but this sensation was somehow different and frightening. Unwilling to admit that he was scared or that the nagging pressure was growing worse, he decided to wait it out.

Eleanor peered over her magazine when Bob came back. "You look a little tired," she said. "Why don't we both turn in for the night?"

"I'm OK," he replied. "You go ahead. I just need to belch but can't quite make it. I think I'll take something to settle my stomach. As soon as it goes away, I'll be in."

Quickly downing a bromide, Bob sat down on the couch with a newspaper. Within a few minutes he felt a thin layer of perspiration on his forehead. As he drew his handkerchief across his forehead, he thought about his father's fatal heart attack at age sixty-one. It came as a complete surprise to the family because his father had no history of heart problems. Two years later, his father's brother Roy suffered a mild heart attack, living only four more years before dying of a second attack in his sleep.

Fighting back his anxiety, Bob tried to reassure himself. "I hardly eat any saturated fat," he thought, "My cholesterol is low; I haven't smoked in years. I could lose a little weight, and my blood pressure may be a little high, but overall I'm in good shape."

He settled back with his newspaper, but the feeling of pressure in his chest was getting worse, and his growing sense of fear made it hard to concentrate. Finally, a few minutes after midnight he went into the bedroom.

"Eleanor," he said, grim faced, "I know this sounds crazy, but I think I'm having a heart attack."

Instantly awake, Eleanor bolted upright. She gasped when she saw Bob standing by the side of the bed, pale as gray-tinged ice.

In the emergency room, a physician questioned and examined the frightened man, then ordered an electrocardiogram and a blood sample. Although the tests were inconclusive (several hours may pass before tests can confirm a heart attack), the doctor kept Bob in the coronary care unit overnight to monitor his heart, and repeated the tests in the morning.

Then Bob received the terrifying news: he had indeed suffered a heart attack. No longer fearful, Bob was incredulous—and angry. "Maybe I don't exercise enough and I've gained a few pounds, but I religiously follow a low-fat diet. How could I have had a heart attack?"

The doctor could only shrug, saying, "I really don't know. Some people, lots of them, eat what should be healthy diets and have normal cholesterols, but still have heart attacks."

Neither the patient, his wife nor his doctor knew that Bob was a victim of Syndrome X, a silent condition that often triggers "the heart attack that shouldn't have happened."

THE "UNKNOWN" PROBLEM WITH A PARADOXICAL SOLUTION

There's good news and bad news in the battle against heart disease. The good news is that thanks to better methods of diagnosis, plus new drugs and surgical techniques, we can detect heart disease much sooner than ever, relieve chest pain and shortness of breath related to heart disease, bypass clogged coronary arteries, effectively treat people who have survived heart attacks and even, in some cases, stop a heart attack in progress.

The bad news is that despite these tremendous technical advances, despite emphasizing good nutrition for two decades, despite lowering our cholesterol levels and cutting fat from our diets, we're still likely to develop heart disease and die of heart attacks. Heart disease remains the number-one killer in this country. Millions will fall prey to a fatal heart attack, many dying without any warning whatsoever. Every 20 seconds, someone, somewhere in America, has a heart attack. And every 34 seconds, someone dies of heart disease. Why? We have powerful drugs to lower cholesterol; high-tech coronary care units place tremendous amounts of technology at the disposal of doctors treating heart patients; triple and quadruple bypass surgeries to restore blood flow to the heart are now routine. Most everyone knows they should protect their hearts by eating a low-fat, high-carbohydrate diet, and exercising regularly—and many of us do. Why, then, are so many of us still dropping dead of heart attacks?

The problem lies in a little-known but very common metabolic disorder called Syndrome X. If you have Syndrome X, your coronary arteries are under attack. These arteries, which bring fresh blood to your heart muscle, are being "cut" and "wounded," are filling with "scabs" and cellular debris, are slowly being dammed up and closed off. This quiet malady's most direct effect is to interfere with the ability of insulin to move glucose (sugar) into certain cells for later use. Unknown millions of heart attacks have been caused by the failure of insulin, the body's "sugar cop," to do its job. This means that, for tens of millions of people, cholesterol is not the underlying problem leading to heart disease. And that's why, if you have Syndrome X, simply lowering your total cholesterol or LDL "bad" cholesterol is not enough to shield you from a heart attack.

Even stranger, to most people, is the idea that one way to guard against Syndrome X is to ignore the "best" medical advice, to shun the low-fat, high-carbohydrate diet everyone "knows" is good for the heart. If you have Syndrome X—and 60–75 million Americans do—that "good" diet can be deadly. If you have the syndrome, carefully dieting to lower your total cholesterol or LDL cholesterol won't solve the problem. In fact, conscientiously doing so may make a heart attack even more likely.

The Number-One Predictor of Heart Disease

Syndrome X, also known as the "insulin resistance syndrome," may be the surest route to a heart attack. It is as powerful a predictor of coronary heart disease as elevated cholesterol or LDL "bad" cholesterol, if not more so.

We don't know exactly how many hearts have been attacked by Syndrome X, although it may be responsible for as many as 50 percent of all heart attacks—or even more. Unfortunately, very few people are aware of Syndrome X, know whether or not they have it or are doing anything about it. And their doctors aren't telling them.

WHAT IS SYNDROME X?

This deadly heart ailment begins in the bloodstream, shortly after we eat. That's not a startling idea, for we know that eating fatty or cholesterol-laden foods can be bad for our hearts. However, the Syndrome X culprit isn't red meat or butter, it's carbohydrates. Yet these carbohydrates are reluctant, inadvertent offenders.

Before entering the body proper, our food is broken down into various constituent parts in the intestine. One of these is glucose (blood sugar) from carbohydrates. Upon entering our cells, some of the glucose is put right to work providing the energy that cells need to perform their various tasks. The rest is stored in certain cells for later use. But the glucose doesn't simply flow into the storage cells. Instead, it must be guided in by insulin, a protein secreted by the pancreas.

Insulin acts like a shepherd, herding its precious flock into the cellular "corrals." Unfortunately, in many of us, glucose behaves like a group of errant sheep, stubbornly refusing to go where the shepherd directs. When that happens, the pancreas pumps out more and more insulin. That's the biochemical equivalent of sending out more and more "shepherds" to get the "sheep" into the "corrals." Imagine hundreds of shepherds chasing thousands of sheep across a pristine field covered with thick, beautiful green grass. Those hundreds of feet and thousands of hoofs will quickly tear up the field, ripping out or flattening down clumps of grass. Soon, the field that once looked so green and lush will be trampled and scarred, brown and dirty.

Something similar happens inside your body when glucose refuses to move into the storage cells at insulin's command. The interior linings of your arteries, like the grassy field, are "ripped" and "trampled" as the body attempts to overcome this problem.

Eventually, the insulin "shepherds" corral the glucose, and order is restored in the body. But all is not well, for the "field" (the lining of your coronary arteries) is damaged, and there's other damage, as well. This damage sets the stage for heart disease.

It's Not Always Necessary, Yet It's Vital

Not all cells need insulin in order to absorb blood sugar. Brain cells, for example, do so without the help of the hormone. It's as if evolution realized that getting fuel (glucose) into brain cells was too important a task to depend on the presence of insulin at the right time, in the right amounts. Kidney and red blood cells also "grab" the glucose they need without insulin's assistance. On the other hand, muscle and fat (adipose) cells depend on insulin's aid, and that's where the problems with insulin resistance arise.

Excess insulin in the bloodstream prompts the damage associated with Syndrome X, but the insulin is only trying to do its job. The underlying problem is *insulin resistance.* About 25 to 30 percent of Americans are resistant to their own insulin—their "shepherds" are simply not strong enough to properly herd glucose. This means that greater amounts of insulin are required to get the job done. Unfortunately, excess insulin is the first in a series of events which triggers the damage to arteries that may precipitate a heart attack.

Insulin resistance is at the heart of Syndrome X. That's why simply lowering total cholesterol or LDL "bad" cholesterol won't solve the problem. And that's why the low-fat, high-carbohydrate diet so highly recommended by most physicians and health organizations is so dangerous for those with the disorder. Remember, carbohydrates become glucose, and glucose *must* be herded into certain cells. That requires insulin. More carbohydrate equals more glucose equals more insulin: that's the formula for disaster for those with this "unknown" syndrome.

Up until about ten years ago, insulin resistance was recognized as a malady which, if not compensated for, could lead to type 2 diabetes. Thanks to thirty years' worth of research into Syndrome X, we now know that even if you never develop diabetes, you can still suffer other ill effects from insulin resistance and high insulin levels: you may suffer from a constellation of changes that greatly increases your risk of coronary heart disease. In short, if you are insulin resistant, you are in real trouble.

WHO IS LIKELY TO DEVELOP SYNDROME X?

Syndrome X is not an exotic disease visited on a few genetically unlucky people. Between 60 and 75 million of us are insulin resistant. A small percent of those millions, perhaps 5 to 10 percent, will develop Type 2 diabetes because their pancreases simply can't produce enough insulin to overcome the insulin resistance. The pancreases of the remaining people will furiously secrete insulin until the resistance is overcome, thus setting the stage for heart disease.

Although we haven't yet mapped out all the genes responsible for triggering Syndrome X, we do know that there must be abnormalities in several genes before the disease can manifest itself. We also know that ethnicity plays a role, with people of non-European origin being at a much greater risk.

Family history also factors into the equation, with your odds of developing Syndrome X increasing substantially if you have a family history of diseases related to insulin resistance, such as heart attack, hypertension and type 2 diabetes. Lifestyle factors are apparently as important as the genetic: improper diet, obesity, lack of physical activity and cigarette smoking worsen Syndrome X. The fact that our behavior plays a role in the syndrome is good and bad news. We can't alter our genetic heritage, but we *can* change our diets and daily habits.

The Difference Between Syndrome X and Diabetes

Problems with insulin are at the heart of both Syndrome X and type 2 diabetes.

If you have type 2 diabetes, your insulin isn't working well; it's not as effective as it should be. When sugar (glucose) from food enters your bloodstream, your pancreas does its best to secrete enough insulin to overcome the insulin resistance and escort that glucose into certain body cells. If the pancreas cannot keep up the effort, the amount of sugar in your blood will continue to rise until there's so much, it begins entering the cells by sheer force. When this happens, you have type 2 diabetes. All that excess glucose in your bloodstream causes damage that can lead to blindness, kidney failure and other problems.

Something similar happens with Syndrome X: the insulin pumped out by your pancreas isn't able to guide glucose into designated cells properly. But—and this is the key difference—with Syndrome X your pancreas shifts into high gear, spewing out more and more insulin until all the glucose has been safely tucked into the cells.

The difference between Syndrome X and type 2 diabetes is that people with the former can continue pumping out the large amounts of insulin needed to use glucose normally, while those with type 2 diabetes cannot. Being able to produce enough insulin to overcome insulin resistance keeps your blood sugar from going too high, so you don't suffer from type 2 diabetes and its many ills. That's the good news.

Unfortunately, you're left with very high levels of insulin in your bloodstream, concentrations that lead to the many risk factors for Syndrome X and heart disease. And, to make matters worse, the ability of your pancreas to manufacture insulin may weaken over time, adding type 2 diabetes to your list of ailments.

THE NEWEST, MOST IMPORTANT RISK FACTOR

Thanks to decades' worth of painstaking study and observation, physicians have compiled a list of the risk factors for heart disease. That list usually looks likes this:

- Elevated LDL "bad" cholesterol
- Low HDL "good" cholesterol
- Obesity

- Elevated blood pressure
- Diabetes mellitus
- Cigarette smoking
- Lack of physical activity

The more of these risk factors you have, the greater your odds of suffering a heart attack.

This standard list of heart disease risk factors is a good start, but it's missing a vital ingredient. The list is inadequate for those with Syndrome X because it does not address insulin resistance or compensatory hyperinsulinemia (excess insulin) and their consequences.

The complete list of heart disease risk factors for people with Syndrome X looks like this:

Syndrome X risk factors
- Impaired glucose tolerance
- High insulin levels (hyperinsulinemia)
- Elevated triglycerides (blood fats)
- Low HDL "good" cholesterol
- Slow clearance of fat from the blood (exaggerated postprandial lipemia)
- Smaller, more dense LDL "bad" cholesterol particles
- Increased propensity of the blood to form clots
- Decreased ability to dissolve blood clots
- Elevated blood pressure

Lifestyle factors that worsen Syndrome X
- Obesity
- Lack of physical activity
- The wrong diet
- Cigarette smoking

The additional independent risk factor:
- Higher than normal LDL cholesterol

Notice the differences. The Syndrome X heart disease risk factor list includes the rate at which fat clears from the blood, not just the amount of fat in the blood. It also considers the formation and clearance of blood clots, and the physical characteristics of LDL cholesterol (not just the amount).

Just how important are the Syndrome X risk factors? Several studies have shown that a low HDL cholesterol, a central feature of Syndrome X, is at least as powerful, if not more so, in increasing risk of heart attack as is high LDL cholesterol. Studies have shown that every separate component of Syndrome X is an individually significant heart attack risk factor. That means that the more components of Syndrome X you have, the greater the heart attack risk. The most reputable research studies reflect this profound fact. For example, the Quebec Cardiovascular Study found that for each 30 percent elevation in insulin levels, there was a 70 percent increase in risk of heart disease over a five-year period. The risk increased with each added component of Syndrome X.

THERE IS A SOLUTION

The best way to prevent Syndrome X is to choose your parents carefully. After all, if you have a family history of heart attack, you run a greater risk of having one yourself. But since the wonders of modern biology have yet to give us the option of choosing our parents, we must find a more practical solution.

There are numerous heart attack prevention programs and diets. But none of them gives you the complete and effective approach that attacks *all* risk factors simultaneously, for none deals with Syndrome X and insulin resistance. In fact, much of their dietary advice makes the syndrome decidedly worse.

The solution to Syndrome X is based on rigorous scientific research. It is safe, effective and very easy to follow. The dietary changes require only slight adaptations for most people, who are delighted to learn that the Syndrome X Diet™ allows significantly more fat than the standard "heart healthy" diet. This means that your health-enhancing diet actually tastes good! Since it's nutritionally balanced, all family members can share the same food, even if they don't have the disorder. The nondietary facets of the program are equally practical and easy to do.

Syndrome X is a complicated disorder, making it impossible to devise a magical "one size fits all" cure. Nonetheless, it's relatively easy to identify your practical needs and the ideal solution. Your particular strategy will be based on your laboratory results.

Which strategy you adopt depends on how many aspects of Syndrome X you have, and how severe they are. It's possible to have developed all aspects of Syndrome X, or only one or two. Some people suffer from all the manifestations at severe levels, some develop one or two at a slight level and others land somewhere in between. The more Syndrome X risk factors you have, and the more severe they are, the greater your risk of having a heart attack. But even if you are only standing on the precipice of Syndrome X, adopting and maintaining a preventive program now will greatly enhance your heart health for the rest of your life.

Having a safe and effective plan for yourself has psychological as well as physical benefits. Imagine waking up each morning feeling as if you were going to live a long and productive life. You take a brisk half-hour walk feeling as if you can tackle anything that comes your way. You eat a healthy breakfast that satisfies you until lunch. At work you focus easily as you knock off tasks one by one. At night you float off to sleep, as sure as anyone can be that your good fortune will continue. Why so confident? Because you've been tested for Syndrome X and you know you have it. But you are following the prevention program and have the problem well under control. You are on your way to preventing the damage to your coronary arteries caused by the syndrome. Things have never looked better.

This scenario is quite realistic. There's no magic to it. Anyone can undergo the simple diagnostic tests for the syndrome, and anyone can get treatment. If you know what to look for, Syndrome X can be easily identified and effectively treated.

WHEN THE HEART
IS UNDER SIEGE

LUB-DUB. LUB-DUB. LUB-DUB. LUB-DUB. Faster than once a second your heart sounds the double beat that signifies it is working, pumping blood through your body. "Lub," the first part of the double beat, is heard when the heart valves open, allowing blood to enter. The second sound, "dub," chimes in as the valves close behind the blood that has just left the heart.

It's the drumbeat of life, sounding some 60 to 80 times a minute, 100,000 times a day, over two and one-half billion times a lifetime. But it's a lone drummer carrying the entire load. If the regular rhythm becomes erratic, if the pace speeds or slows too much, or if it ceases entirely for even a brief period of time, you may die. And, in fact, many of us do die when our hearts stop beating regularly, strongly. Worldwide, 12 million of us fall victim to heart disease every year; that's nearly 23 every minute. Heart disease is the greatest killer of all, claiming more lives than stroke, cancer, accidents, pneumonia or diabetes.

Heart Disease by the Numbers

According to the American Heart Association, there are over 1 million new and "repeat" heart attacks per year, and close to half a million people die from heart attacks annually. Approximately 14 million currently living Americans have had heart attacks, angina (chest pain) or other manifestations of coronary heart disease.

THE FOUR-CHAMBERED PUMP

For many scientific investigators, the workings of the human brain and the secrets of our genes stir the most excitement, and research in these areas holds the promise of the greatest cures. To them, the heart is a little on the dull side—vital, but not terribly exciting. After all, they might say, it's just a glorified pump.

Ah, but what a pump. With every double beat it squirts out about two and one-half ounces of blood. That adds up to five to six quarts every minute, or an amazing 1,800 to 2,160 *gallons* a day. Imagine 2,000 gallons of milk; that's enough to fill sixty or seventy refrigerators, and that's how much your heart pumps throughout your body every day of your life, without fail.

It all begins when "used" blood from all over your body returns to your heart, specifically to the right side of the heart. Spilling out of the giant vena cava veins, this blood flows into the heart's upper right chamber, called the right atrium. It's a small chamber, a little waiting area where the blood pauses for just a moment. Then the muscular walls of the atrium contract and the blood drops down through the tricuspid valve into the right ventricle. Larger and more powerfully muscled than the atrium above, the right ventricle shoots the "used" blood completely out of the heart and to the lungs, where it exchanges its carbon dioxide for a fresh supply of oxygen. Then the newly oxygenated fluid returns to the heart, this time to the left side.

There it flows into the left atrium, another small "waiting room" where it waits briefly before the muscular walls squeeze inward, the mitral valve opens and the blood is pumped into the left ventricle below. This is the mightiest of the heart's four chambers. Its muscles are the thickest, making it the most powerful pumping chamber. When it squeezes, "fresh" blood shoots out into the aorta, the great artery arching out of and away from the heart. Once in the aorta, the richly oxygenated blood travels through a network of increasingly smaller vessels to every part of the body. Eventually the blood returns, via the two vena cava veins, to begin the process again.

It's easy to remember: the heart is essentially a large muscle with four chambers. The two atriums are the smaller "waiting rooms" above, the two ventricles are the larger, stronger "pumping stations" below. The right side of the heart collects "used" blood and sends it to the lungs, the left side gathers oxygenated blood from the lungs and sends it out to the body. Upper, lower, left and right, the four chambers work in concert, constantly sounding the double beat of life. Over a lifetime, each of the two ventricles will squirt out some 150,000 tons of blood. To do so, they must generate a force equal to that necessary to raise 10 tons, 10 miles into the air.

Charging the Heart

Ever wonder what makes your heart tick? Electricity. A specialized bundle of tissue in the right atrium, the upper right chamber of the heart, sends out electrical signals that keep the heart muscle beating. If something interferes with the proper flow of electricity through the heart, you may suffer from irregular heartbeats, called arrhythmias. If the arrhythmias are serious, doctors may implant a pacemaker to keep your heart beating regularly. Modern, battery-powered pacemakers can keep a heart beating steadily for up to ten years.

A CROWN OF ARTERIES

Propelled out of the left ventricle, "fresh" blood enters the giant aorta, the first of a series of arterial "roadways" that take it to both near and distant parts of the body, where it will deliver its load of oxygen. Almost immediately, a small portion of this blood is diverted, doubling back into the heart muscle itself, via the arteries known as the coronary arteries. It's this part of the heart—the heart muscle, not the chambers—and this relatively small portion of blood that we're concerned with when we talk about heart disease, specifically coronary heart disease, or a heart attack.

The heart is a powerful muscle. Like any other muscle, body part or cell, it must receive a continuous supply of "fresh" blood, else it will soon die. You wouldn't think this is a problem. After all, the heart is awash with blood; all the blood in the body continually circulates through it. But the heart muscle can't use the blood flowing in and out of its four chambers; that blood is off limits. The heart muscle has its own, specially designated supply of blood diverted from the aorta and into the coronary arteries.

So named because the larger ones seem to sit like a crown on the heart's surface, the coronary arteries tunnel into the heart muscle, into the chamber walls themselves to bring oxygen-rich blood to the heart muscle. And blood flows through the heart muscle just as it does through any muscle. It begins in the coronary arteries, then flows into smaller arterioles. From there it moves into the tiny capillaries, where it surrenders its oxygen and takes up waste products to carry away. Having discharged its duty, the blood begins the return trip, moving into the small venules, then the larger veins. Eventually it makes its way to the giant vena cava, the large vein carrying "used" blood back to the heart, where it mixes with blood coming from other parts of the body. It joins the blood pool, which drops into the right atrium, and begins moving through the four chambers.

But what happens if the flow of blood through the tiny coronary arteries or arterioles is blocked? Depending on which artery is blocked, to what degree and for how long, the result can range from unnoticeable to deadly.

DAMMING THE FLOW

Think about the plumbing in your house: a series of pipes tunnel through the walls, carrying "fresh" water into your kitchen and bathrooms, and "used" water away. The water comes from the city supply into your house through a wide pipe, then goes through smaller ones until it reaches its final destination.

Suppose a tiny rubber ball somehow got into the city water supply, drifting through the large pipes until, by chance, it got into your plumbing. It wouldn't matter at first, for the pipe carrying water from the water main into your house is nice and wide; the ball would simply flow in with the water. And nothing much would happen as the water carried the small ball into the narrower pipes in your walls, for they're wide enough to accommodate the necessary water and the ball. But eventually the ball would be carried into a very narrow pipe, where it would get stuck. Then there would be trouble, for water could no longer flow through that little pipe. All the other plumbing in your house would work well, but this one pipe would be dammed up. No water could get through. All the faucets "downstream" of the ball-dam would quickly dry up.

Something similar happens in the coronary arteries. The water main is your aorta, the large artery in which "fresh" blood begins its journey; the smaller pipes are the coronary arteries and arterioles; the house is your heart muscle; the ball is plaque. For various reasons plaque may grow in the arteries, creating a dam. Then heart muscle "downstream" of the dam "dries up" and dies, although portions of the heart muscle supplied by other arteries and arterioles are un-harmed.

Doctors call this a "coronary," "coronary incident," "coronary event," "coronary thrombosis," "coronary occlusion" or "myocardial infarct," although almost everyone else refers to it as a heart attack. If the problem strikes in a relatively insignificant coronary artery (an "outlying" pipe supplying blood to a small area of heart tissue), the damage may be slight. But if the blood flow is dammed in an impor-tant part of the heart's plumbing, an artery feeding a larger section of heart muscle, the consequences can be deadly.

TWO WAYS TO BLOCK THE FLOW

The human body, of course, is much more complex than home plumb-ing. It would be impossible to fully explain all of the "hows and whys" of blockages in the coronary arteries because, frankly, we doc-tors don't have all the answers. We understand the general outlines and many of the details, but we haven't yet fully mapped out the en-tire process, so we can't answer every question.

This much we do know. The building of "arterial dams" is a com-plex process involving the interior lining of the arteries, certain im-mune system cells, blood fat, cholesterol and other substances in the blood. In general terms, the unfortunate building process begins when the interior lining of a coronary artery is damaged. Something floating in the blood nicks, scratches or rips the lining—just a little bit, that's all it takes.

What is to blame for the arterial injuries? For many years, LDL "bad" cholesterol has been considered the chief culprit. Recently, some researchers have begun pointing the finger at an amino acid called homocysteine. And, as we'll see in the next chapter, Syndrome X is responsible for a great deal of the trouble.

Whatever the cause, the stage has been set. Sensing damage, cer-tain cells called monocytes hurry to the scene, triggering a series of complex events as the body tries to repair the damage. Soon the scratch is knitted shut, but at a cost. A little "scar," a tiny "over-growth" marks the spot where the damage occurred. We call the scar tissue plaque, and it sits like a little "mound" on the interior lining of the artery, jutting out into the bloodstream. Just as a little pile of rocks, twigs, leaves, bottles, cans and other debris sitting on the bottom of a river slightly upsets the flow of water, the little "plaque mound" pro-trudes into the bloodstream, causing a little turbulence. It's not a seri-ous problem—not yet.

Over time, more and more "debris" floats by and "sticks" to the little plaque mound. LDL "bad" cholesterol, blood fat, more immune system cells and other substances pile on top, causing the mound to grow. Many years will likely pass before the slowly growing pile of plaque causes any problem. At some point, however, it will grow from a little mound into a major blockage. Enough blood will still flow by to keep heart tissue nourished, but it will be getting close to the cutoff point.

Then one of two things can happen. The plaque dam may grow to the point where the flow of blood is severely hampered, slowed to a trickle. Heart muscle "downstream" may scream in pain as it's slowly starved of nourishment. Or the dam "wall" may suddenly rupture, al-lowing the gunk in the dam to pour into the bloodstream and trigger a clot. If that happens, the damaged artery will slam shut, abruptly turning off the faucet. Consider yourself lucky if your heart gives you early warning by sending out pain signals—there's probably enough time to get to your doctor's office and begin a heart-healthy program. But if the blood flow is suddenly stopped by the abrupt closure of an artery, and if this happens in an important coronary artery, the first warning pain in your chest may be the last thing you ever feel.

ATHEROSCLEROSIS

Atherosclerosis is the word we use to describe the mound-forming damage to arteries that can lead to a heart attack. Everyone develops some degree of atherosclerosis as they grow older, although the extent of the damage and how rapidly it occurs varies widely. In the early 1950s, autopsies on young American and Korean soldiers killed dur-ing the Korean War showed that the process was much more ad-vanced in the American men than in their Korean counterparts. Since then we've learned that diet, exercise habits, heredity and other fac-tors—including Syndrome X—are all linked to atherosclerosis.

The word atherosclerosis comes from a Greek word meaning "gruel." That's an apt description of the deposits in arteries. If you peer into a microscope at an artery taken from someone with advanced coronary heart disease, you can see the fat and cell components "growing" out of the artery wall. If you run your finger across the deposits, they'll feel hard and crusty; some areas of the artery wall will have cracked open and leaked blood. But this condition didn't happen all at once. Atherosclerosis typically starts in early adulthood, long before a heart attack strikes.

Which Is Which?

You've undoubtedly heard people speaking about both atherosclerosis and arteriosclerosis. Although most laypeople—and even some physicians—use the words interchangeably, they do have different definitions.

Arteriosclerosis, the more general term, refers to thickening of the walls and loss of elasticity in small and mid-sized arteries. When arteries lose their elasticity, the flow of blood may falter.

Atherosclerosis is a more specific form of arteriosclerosis characterized by the buildup of the plaque "mounds" on the artery walls. It may be caused by various factors, including elevated blood fats, high blood pressure, diabetes and Syndrome X.

Much of what accounts for a higher risk of heart attack in one person than in another is the rate at which the atherosclerotic process advances. Several factors have been linked to the problem in varying degrees, including elevated LDL "bad" cholesterol in the blood, low levels of HDL "good" cholesterol, high blood pressure, diabetes, obesity, a sedentary lifestyle and cigarette smoking. Syndrome X is a "new" risk factor, at least as dangerous as the others. In someone with Syndrome X, the atherosclerotic process races ahead, piling more and more "debris" on the plaque dam and dramatically increasing the odds of an early blockage and sudden death.

Fortunately, heart attacks are not always fatal. In fact, only about one-third are deadly. Getting immediate treatment during a heart attack can be lifesaving: with modern drugs and technology, some serious attacks can be stopped in their tracks. If you notice any of these symptoms of an impending or progressing heart attack, get help immediately: heavy pressure or chest pain lasting more than a few min-

---

Coronary Artery Disease Versus Heart Attack

Coronary refers to the heart, so coronary artery disease refers to problems with the arteries that carry "fresh" blood to the heart muscle. More specifically, coronary artery disease is atherosclerosis, the buildup of plaque that disrupts the flow of blood to the heart muscle and may eventually trigger a heart attack. You can have coronary artery disease without suffering a heart attack, if the disease does not progress too far. Some people survive despite a great deal of coronary artery disease, with key coronary arteries blocked 50, 60, even 70 percent.

---

utes; shortness of breath or difficulty breathing; chest pain moving into the shoulder, arm, back or jaw; heart palpitations (irregular heartbeat); prolonged stomach or upper abdominal pain; faintness, nausea or vomiting; intense perspiration or cold sweat; unexplained anxiety, weakness or fatigue; unusual paleness.

Having these symptoms does not necessarily mean that you're having a heart attack. But if they do strike, call your physician or go to an emergency room right away. A heart attack is a serious problem; it's better to be safe than sorry. If you are having an attack, the sooner treatment begins, the better.

A doctor will probably begin assessing you by discussing your medical and personal history and performing a physical examination. She may also ask what you were doing when the symptoms began and so forth, looking for clues to suggest the cause of your distress. (Heartburn, for example, can cause severe chest pain.) She will also likely run an EKG (electrocardiogram) to look for evidence of ischemia (lack of blood flow to the heart muscle) and draw blood to check for the presence of certain enzymes that only appear in the blood in large amounts following a heart attack.

What happens next varies. If you are having a heart attack and if the emergency room or hospital has the appropriate technology and expertise, you may be given immediate fibrinolytic therapy. With this high-tech "heart attack stopper," medicine is infused into either your veins or coronary arteries to dissolve the blood clot causing the attack before much more heart muscle dies. If it appears that you have already suffered a heart attack, or if that possibility can't be ruled out, you will be admitted to the coronary care unit for monitoring and possible intervention. The doctor may call for a coronary arteriogram to check for narrowing or blockages in your coronary arteries, or perhaps angioplasty to "pump up" a narrowed artery. If there's no evidence that you are now suffering or have recently suffered a heart attack, you may be sent home and advised to make an appointment with your personal physician for a more thorough evaluation.

Is All Heart Disease a "Heart Attack"?

Heart attack is the most common form of heart disease, but it isn't the only problem afflicting our internal pumps. Other ailments include:

- Problems with the heart valves, such as rheumatic heart disease or mitral valve prolapse.
- An inflammation of the thin sac covering the heart, called pericarditus.
- An inflammation of the heart's inner lining, called endocarditis.
- Heart failure, the inability of the heart to continue pumping steadily and vigorously. This may be result of a previous heart attack or can be triggered by elevated blood pressure.
- Cardiomyopathy, a condition in which heart muscle is partially replaced by fibrous tissue that cannot keep the blood flowing properly. It may be caused by alcohol, medications, viruses, bacteria, metabolic errors and other problems.

Four chambers, an electrical "triggering" mechanism, fluid flowing through the chambers and the heart muscle itself: the human heart is indeed a wondrous, marvelous instrument. With the proper care, it can keep ticking, and keep you kicking, for a lifetime.

NEW HOPE FROM

AN UNLIKELY SOURCE

IN 1968, MY COLLEAGUES and I at Stanford University published the first studies showing that:

- it is possible to measure the degree to which muscle cells utilize blood sugar (glucose) when stimulated by a protein hormone called insulin;
- insulin's ability to do its job varies wildly from person to person (the less effective your insulin, the more insulin-resistant you are);
- most people who are insulin resistant are capable of producing large amounts of insulin in order to compensate and force glucose out of the bloodstream and into the cells that need it for nourishment;
- if insulin-resistant people cannot produce enough insulin to overcome the resistance, they develop type 2 diabetes.

The scientific world did not stand up to applaud, possibly because these findings ran contrary to what doctors of the time absolutely "knew" to be true. In the forty-five years since insulin had been discovered, medical scientists came to believe that the only insulin consideration was how much of it the body could make, and that the less made, the higher the blood sugar would go and the greater the degree of diabetes. The possibility that there could be something wrong with the way insulin worked in some people and that their bodies had to secrete large amounts of it to overcome the problem were completely foreign ideas. The idea of insulin resistance didn't make sense to the medical establishment.

Despite the lack of peer support, I continued studying the ways that the body uses and responds to insulin. After twenty additional years of study and observation, I published the first paper showing that insulin-resistant individuals were at great risk of developing what I named Syndrome X, a cluster of abnormalities that is a major (albeit "unknown") cause of heart disease.

An Ancient Substance, Newly Recognized

Hundreds of millions of years ago, life on Earth consisted of a sea of single-cell organisms. Out of this primordial soup—we may never know exactly when—insulin emerged as a primary growth factor for cell multiplication. Insulin and insulin-like molecules attached themselves to receptors on the cells, gave them the signal to start multiplying and then told them when to stop. However, insulin's "duties" evolved to the point that the dogfish shark, a primitive, boneless creature that arrived on the scene long ago, had a pancreas that secretes digestive juices containing a primitive form of insulin.

It wasn't until 1923 that we discovered insulin and began to explore its duties in the body—and learned how to keep diabetics alive. In modern man, this hormone is no longer needed as a primary growth factor; it doesn't tell cells when to start and stop multiplying. Instead, it focuses on shuttling blood sugar into the appropriate cells, where it's used for energy. Sixty-five years after the discovery of insulin, I described the cluster of abnormalities tied to insulin resistance and high levels of insulin in the blood that encourage heart disease, naming it Syndrome X. We now know that too much insulin can be just as dangerous as too little.

THE INSULIN IMPERATIVE

Insulin is not a villain, not a rogue hormone or the "hidden" cause of untold diseases. Instead, it's a naturally occurring hormone produced by specialized cells in the pancreas called beta cells, or B-cells for short. We need insulin, in the right amounts, at the right times, to stay alive. And it's usually present just when we need it, in exactly the proper amount. Where Syndrome X is concerned, there's nothing wrong with the insulin itself or the insulin-producing parts of the pancreas. The problem has to do with the abnormal way in which the body responds to that insulin.

Simply put, insulin is a protein hormone that regulates the flow of energy throughout the body. It's the "door opener" that allows blood sugar to flow into specialized body cells, where it's used for energy. Your body needs a continual supply of energy, day and night, whether you're active or not, awake or asleep. Since you need energy at all times, insulin must always be present in the blood to help blood sugar get through those "doors" and into designated body cells.

A Little-Known Organ

The pancreas, a long organ sitting in your mid-abdomen, plays an important role in processing food. Most of the pancreas is filled with cells that have nothing to do with insulin. Instead, they release digestive enzymes directly into the small intestine, where they break down the fat, protein and carbohydrate in your food into small particles your body can absorb for energy. But even as the digestive enzymes are working, your pancreas is revving up your insulin-secreting system.

If most pancreatic cells release digestive enzymes, where does insulin come from? This mystery was solved before we knew what insulin was, and what it did. In the late nineteenth century, a German pathologist named Paul Langerhans realized that concentrated pools of cells were scattered throughout the pancreas. These clusters, named the islets of Langerhans, contain four different types of cells, each releasing a different kind of hormone into the bloodstream. Nearly 90 percent of the cells in your islets of Langerhans are beta cells, which secrete insulin.

While pancreatic enzymes act only on the food in your intestine, pancreatic hormones such as insulin get into your bloodstream and travel throughout your body. This ability to spread far and wide allows insulin to regulate the activity of cells throughout your body.

Before you eat your breakfast in the morning, the energy you need to keep your heart beating, your muscles working and thoughts forming—in short, the energy needed to keep you alive—is provided by glucose from your liver cells, amino acids from muscle cells and fatty acids from fat cells. (With no "new" energy coming in by way of food, your body has to draw on its stores.) Your pancreas aids in the process by continually secreting just enough insulin to make sure the energy is used properly. Without this system of storing and releasing energy, you wouldn't be able to get out of bed in the morning. You couldn't even lift an eyelid.

Shortly after you eat breakfast, the system goes into reverse as your body, awash with "new" energy from food, processes and then stores it away. The switch begins as the digestive products of your food—particularly glucose derived from carbohydrates and amino acids from protein—stimulate your pancreas to release more insulin. Naturally, your blood insulin levels rise. Your liver stops releasing glucose for energy, instead storing it as glycogen. Your muscle cells use newly absorbed glucose and amino acids as they rebuild themselves and prepare to provide the energy your muscles will need later, when you're not eating. Your fat cells store newly absorbed fat for later use. As the process winds down, your pancreas cuts back on insulin production. Two or three hours after the meal, your blood insulin levels are back to where they started.

All through the day and night, your pancreas releases insulin—more or less, depending on your needs. After you've eaten, the pancreas sends out a lot of this hormone to "corral" the excess blood sugar from your food and store it in the proper cells. At night, when your liver is releasing a steady but small supply of blood sugar in response to lesser needs, a relatively small amount of insulin comes from the pancreas to open the cellular doors for that glucose.

Normally, the digestive and insulin-secreting processes run smoothly, keeping your blood sugar concentration within a narrow range while efficiently regulating your energy needs and usage. In order to keep the process going without a hitch, your pancreas must secrete extra insulin quickly when it's demanded. And, of course, your muscle, fat and liver cells must respond to the insulin efficiently.

A series of simple feedback loops continually fine-tune the entire operation. Food comes into the body, some of it is converted into blood sugar, and more insulin is released. (How much and what kind of food you eat determines how much insulin must be released.) When there's less blood sugar circulating, less insulin is needed. If everything is working properly, there's always enough insulin to handle the sugar in the blood; the body keeps everything nicely balanced. As long as the pancreas continues pumping out the insulin, everything will be fine. It's that simple—or so we thought.

WHEN SOMETHING GOES WRONG

Our groundbreaking 1968 study showed that it's not as simple as "either the pancreas makes enough insulin or it doesn't." Yes, it's true that insulin must be manufactured and secreted in the right amounts, at the right time. But that's not all there is to it. Your muscle, fat and liver cells have to respond appropriately—and promptly—to that insulin, or problems arise.

Two things can happen when the insulin system breaks down: either you secrete little or no insulin and develop type 1 diabetes, or your pancreas pumps out plenty of insulin but your body doesn't respond to it normally, putting you at risk for either type 2 diabetes or Syndrome X.

- If you manufacture little or no insulin, you will develop type 1 diabetes. Also called insulin-dependent diabetes mellitus, or IDDM, it is a dramatic disease. Fortunately, it's relatively rare. It tends to show up early in life, usually developing in childhood when the immune system mistakenly attacks the pancreas, largely or totally destroying its ability to produce insulin. Without sufficient insulin to usher in the blood sugar, body cells "starve." The only way to keep people with type 1 diabetes alive is to give them the insulin they can no longer manufacture on their own. Only 5 to 10 percent of diabetics have type 1, which has nothing to do with type 2, insulin resistance or Syndrome X. In fact, if people with type 1 diabetes manage to produce a little insulin on their own, their bodies respond to it quite well.

- If your pancreas still can make insulin but your body doesn't respond well to the hormone's commands, you can develop type 2 diabetes. Type 2 diabetes is often confused with type 1. After all, with both diseases patients have high blood sugar levels due to insulin problems. But they're really different diseases with different causes. With type 2 diabetes, the immune system has not gone haywire, it has not turned on the pancreas and destroyed that organ's ability to make insulin. The problem is that the amount of insulin being produced—whether it's a normal amount or even more—isn't enough to "open the doors" to certain body cells; they stop responding to insulin's command to let blood sugar in to serve as raw material for the little cellular energy factories.

In the early stages of type 2 diabetes, before the blood sugar rises to extremely high levels, the body compensates almost perfectly by pumping out more insulin. Your blood sugar is a little high, but not too much so. This may work for a while, but eventually your body "gives up" and loses the ability to release enough insulin to overcome the insulin resistance. When that happens, your blood sugar starts climbing and you have type 2 diabetes. This disease, which afflicts over 100 million people worldwide, can be treated with diet, lifestyle changes and medication. Although not nearly as dramatic as type 1 diabetes, type 2 is the leading cause of kidney failure and new cases of blindness in the United States.

INSULIN RESISTANCE, THE BASIC ABNORMALITY OF TYPE 2 DIABETES

Insulin signals certain cells to "open their doors" to blood sugar by attaching itself to specially designated receptors on the cells' surface. But sometimes the "doors" remain closed because these cells have become insulin resistant; they no longer respond to insulin's instructions. Unable to flow into designated cells, the blood sugar accumulates in the bloodstream

From a normal level of approximately 90 mg/dl,[1] blood sugar may rise to 180, 360, 540, even as high as 720 mg/dl! As the blood becomes more and more "sugary," the beta cells in the pancreas take note, producing extra insulin in an attempt to drive that sugar into the cells and push blood sugar levels back to normal.

It's as if the body is pushing harder and harder, "throwing its shoulder" against the stubborn cellular "doors." It may have to secrete two or three times as much insulin as normal—or more—to force that sugar into the cells. But some of us have bodies that can't do that, we can't make the large amounts of insulin needed. And so the blood sugar remains in the blood until, by sheer "weight," it forces its way in. Sufficient amounts of sugar force their way into the cells, but the excess builds up in the blood and spills over into the urine, prompting a diagnosis of type 2 diabetes. The pancreas is still putting out insulin, and that insulin is present and ready for action. The problem lies in the cells that turn a deaf ear to insulin's command, and in the fact that the pancreas just can't make the huge amounts of insulin needed.

---

[1] This is read as 90 milligrams of glucose per deciliter of plasma.

Many of us, however, can make tremendous amounts of insulin. If the normal amount isn't enough to open the cellular doors, we just keep pumping out more and more, as much as it takes to batter those doors down. Eventually, these huge amounts of insulin force the cells to open up and accept the blood sugar. Blood sugar levels fall to normal, the cells have the energy they need to continue working, and everything seems fine.

Unfortunately, all is not well. The beta cells have performed heroically, but have inadvertently caused as much harm as they've averted. The presence of all that extra insulin may harm the interior linings of the arteries, including the coronary arteries that feed the heart; the excess may also trigger other changes in body chemistry that encourage coronary heart disease. Insulin resistance combined with the body's attempt to solve the problem by spewing out tremendous amounts of insulin, called compensatory hyperinsulinemia, leads to the cluster of abnormalities that comprise Syndrome X.

The difference between type 2 diabetes and Syndrome X can be summed up simply: the key problem leading to type 2 diabetes is insulin resistance coupled with the inability to secrete enough insulin to overcome that resistance. The root of Syndrome X, however, is insulin resistance plus compensatory hyperinsulinemia (extra insulin).

A Variable Situation

Insulin action varies enormously in normal people. In the most insulin-sensitive people, insulin action may be ten times more efficient than in the most insulin resistant. About 25 percent of the nondiabetic population is as insulin resistant as those with type 2 diabetes, and is at risk of developing Syndrome X.

CHANGES IN FAT METABOLISM = INCREASED RISK

Syndrome X is not a disease, like the flu, that attacks certain parts of the body, battles with the immune system and disappears within a few weeks. Instead, it is a simple way to refer to a cluster of changes that encourage the onset and development of heart disease. Let's begin delving into the syndrome by looking at the way it alters fat metabolism.

Just like glucose (sugar), fat from your food must be transported through the bloodstream to various body cells for utilization. The process is relatively easy with glucose, but is much more difficult and complicated than you might imagine with fat. The bloodstream is watery, and fat and water do not mix. If you simply put the fat from food into the watery bloodstream, you won't get the desired result. The only way to get the bloodstream to carry fat is to "package" it in water-soluble transport containers made from protein.

There are four major classes of fat-protein packages, called lipoproteins:

- chylomicrons
- very low-density lipoproteins (VLDL)
- low-density lipoproteins (LDL)
- high-density lipoproteins (HDL)

When you eat, enzymes from the pancreas are secreted directly into the small intestine, where they break down the fat into small particles called fatty acids. The cells lining the small intestine absorb these fatty acids and convert them into triglycerides, or what we usually call blood fat. The intestinal cells also produce small amounts of cholesterol and protein, which combine with the triglycerides to form chylomicrons, fat-soluble "transport vehicles" that can carry the fat through the bloodstream.

A Few Quick Definitions

- Triglycerides are made of three fatty acids attached to a glycerol molecule. ("Tri" means three.) This is the transport and storage form of fat.
- Fatty acids are the building blocks of fat, just as amino acids are the individual units that make up protein. When we say the body uses fat, we mean it's using the individual fatty acids.
- Lipo means fat, so a lipoprotein is made from both fat and protein.
- Very low-density lipoprotein (VLDL), low-density lipoprotein (LDL) and high-density lipoprotein (HDL) are differentiated by how much triglyceride they contain. The more triglyceride within these particles, the less dense they are and the more they "float" when separated out in a rapidly spinning centrifuge. VLDL contains the greatest amount of triglyceride, HDL the least.

As the chylomicrons circulate through the bloodstream, an enzyme called lipoprotein lipase, secreted from the lining of the blood vessel walls, breaks down triglycerides into fatty acids plus glycerol once again. "Liberated" from the chylomicrons, the fatty acids are picked up by the fat cells, converted back to triglycerides and stored for later use. As this process continues, the chylomicrons become relatively triglyceride-poor. Now called chylomicron remnants, they are removed from the bloodstream by the liver. (As you can see, the body is constantly building and breaking down. It breaks down the fat in your food to fatty acids, recombines them to form triglycerides, packages the triglycerides into chylomicrons, takes the triglycerides back out of the chylomicrons, and so on.)

While you're eating and for several hours thereafter, chylomicrons are your major source of triglycerides. When you're not eating, different fat-protein particles called very low-density lipoprotein (VLDL) become the major source of triglyceride-rich lipoprotein.

Made by the liver, VLDL is similar in many respects to chylomicrons. It contains large amounts of triglycerides, and is acted upon by the same enzyme system that breaks the triglycerides in chylomicrons into fatty acids. But there are two important differences between VLDL and chylomicrons. First, fatty acids released from VLDL are taken up primarily by muscle, not fat tissue. Second, some VLDL is converted to LDL. (Just as chylomicrons lose their triglycerides to become chylomicron remnants, VLDL loses its triglycerides to become VLDL remnants. But while the chylomicron remnants are removed from the bloodstream by the liver, a portion of the VLDL remnants are converted into LDL.)

LDL and HDL don't play a role in energy metabolism, but they do factor into the heart attack equation—quite strongly. The higher the blood levels of LDL cholesterol, the more likely it is that an excess amount of cholesterol will be deposited in cells lining the artery walls. HDL has just the opposite effect, apparently removing cholesterol from the same blood vessel walls. You want to have less "bad" LDL cholesterol and more "good" HDL cholesterol because your risk of suffering a heart attack rises when LDL goes up, but drops when HDL rises.

HOW SYNDROME X INCREASES THE RISK OF HEART DISEASE

Syndrome X increases the risk of heart disease by interfering with the way your body uses and reacts to fat and other substances. Here are the seven additional risk factors the syndrome throws into the heart disease equation:

1. Elevated triglycerides (blood fat): The insulin resistance and compensatory high insulin seen with Syndrome X encourage your liver to produce more VLDL. Remember that VLDL is a triglyceride-rich substance: the more you make, the higher your triglyceride level. Having Syndrome X means more VLDL, which leads to more fat floating around in your blood and a greater risk of heart disease.

2. Lower HDL "good" cholesterol: An enzyme called cholesteryl ester transfer protein, or CETP for short, transfers cholesterol from your "good" HDL to your "bad" VLDL, exchanging it for triglyceride. The more VLDL you have in your bloodstream, the more cholesterol CETP transfers from your HDL to your VLDL, and the lower your HDL cholesterol level falls. If you have Syndrome X, your liver will make and release more VLDL than normal, so you'll experience more of this transfer. With less HDL cholesterol and more VLDL cholesterol, your risk of heart disease goes up.

3. Exaggerated postprandial lipemia ("fatty" blood after a meal): Everybody's blood fat level rises after eating a meal containing fat, whether that fat is from a hamburger, a pizza, a glass of milk or an avocado. It takes a while for the fat to clear from the blood because the two triglyceride-rich transport vehicles, the chylomicrons and VLDL, must leave the blood by the same route. With Syndrome X, you already have more VLDL than normal in your blood. This means that your ability to remove newly absorbed chylomicrons is impaired. It's like a freeway during rush hour: once the road is jammed, it takes longer for *all* the cars to exit. In people with Syndrome X, VLDL and chylomicrons, as well as their metabolic by-products (chylomicron remnants and VLDL remnants) are removed more slowly from the plasma. This causes an increase in blood fats following a meal, called postprandial lipemia, which is more pronounced in people with Syndrome X. Unfortunately, having these chylomicrons, VLDL, chylomicron remnants and VLDL remnants in your blood for "extra" amounts of time further increases your risk of heart attack.

4. Smaller, denser LDL: LDL cholesterol particles are smaller in people with Syndrome X. We don't know exactly why; it may be caused by the insulin resistance or the resulting excess of insulin in the bloodstream, or it may be related to the high levels of triglycerides seen with the disorder. Whatever the cause, these smaller, denser LDL "bad" cholesterol particles increase your risk of suffering a heart attack.

It's not only the fat particles in the blood that are affected for the worse by Syndrome X. Other changes occur as well.

5. Excess fibrinogen: When we cut ourselves, an almost instantaneous cascade of events causes the blood to clot in order to prevent excessive bleeding. A substance called fibrinogen plays an important role in this process. Unfortunately, not all blood clots are "good" clots. Spontaneous, unnecessary clots can form in coronary arteries damaged by Syndrome X, stop the flow of blood and trigger a sudden heart attack—and having too much fibrinogen can encourage the formation of these dangerous clots. Having plenty of fibrinogen was undoubtedly a lifesaver in ancient times, when the danger of bleeding to death while battling a wild animal was much greater than the risk of a heart attack at age forty or fifty—especially considering that few people lived that long. Today, however, we're much more likely to die of heart disease than we are to bleed to death, so having too much fibrinogen is risky. Unfortunately, people with Syndrome X have high levels of fibrinogen.

6. Excess PAI-1: Since the body is built on a system of checks and balances, there must be something to counteract the clot-encouraging fibrinogen. After all, once the body has the repair process under way, the initial blood clot is no longer needed. And there has to be a way of quickly dissolving any unnecessary, potentially dangerous clots that form, threatening the heart and other parts of the body.

The clot-removing process, called fibrinolysis, is slowed, in part, by a substance called plasminogen activator inhibitor-1, or PAI-1. The more PAI-1 circulating in the bloodstream, the more difficult it is to dissolve clots. That includes the "good" clots that help when we cut ourselves, as well as the "bad" ones that threaten our heart health. Unfortunately, people with Syndrome X have higher levels of PAI-1, which slows the dissolution of clots that can cause a heart attack. The higher your PAI-1, the more likely it is that you will have a heart attack.

7. Hypertension: Hypertension, or elevated blood pressure, is called the "silent killer" because it has no symptoms. You can't feel the increased pressure in your arteries, so you probably don't know anything is wrong. And unless your doctor catches the problem in time, you may not know anything is wrong until that first heart attack or stroke occurs.

Several studies have made it clear that insulin resistance and compensatory hyperinsulinemia, the hallmarks of Syndrome X, tend to raise blood pressure. For example, four long-term studies[2] of healthy volunteers demonstrated that the higher the insulin levels were at the beginning of the study, the more likely one was to eventually develop hypertension. We also know that first-degree relatives (parent, child, etc.) of people with high blood pressure are more insulin resistant than those without family histories of hypertension. And approximately half of all patients with high blood pressure are insulin resistant, and have one or more components of Syndrome X. Moreover, these individuals are the ones most likely to have a heart attack.

Although linked to Syndrome X, hypertension does not cause the problem. The connection between hypertension and Syndrome X is very new, so many questions remain to be answered. For example, being insulin resistant increases the odds of developing high blood pressure, but not everyone with hypertension has Syndrome X.

This relationship is particularly important when considering why heart attacks continue to be such a problem for people with hypertension, despite the effective anti-hypertensive drugs available. (Remember, half of those with hypertension also have Syndrome X.) It's vital that every healthy-heart program address this association, or we'll continue to see little success in shielding hypertensive patients from heart attack.

IN SUM

These are the seven additional monkey wrenches Syndrome X throws into our healthy heart machinery:

- Elevated triglycerides (blood fats)
- Lower HDL "good" cholesterol

[2] (1) E. T. Skarfors, H. O. Lithell, and I. Selinus. Risk factors for the development of hypertension: a 10-year longitudinal study in middle-aged men. *Journal of Hypertension* 9:217–223, 1991; (2) L. Lissner, C. Bengtsson, K. Kristansson, and H. Wedel. Fasting insulin in relation to subsequent blood pressure changes and hypertension in women. *Hypertension* 20:797–801, 1992; (3) L. Taittonen, M. Uhari, M. Nuutinen, J. Turtinen, T. Pokka, and H. K. Akerblom. Insulin in blood pressure among healthy children. *American Journal of Hypertension* 9:193–199, 1996; (4) O. T. Raitakari, K. V. K. Porkka, T. Rommemaa, M. Uhari, H. K. Akerblom, and J. S. A. Viikari. The role of insulin in clustering of serum lipids and blood pressure in children and adolescents. *Diabetologia* 38:1042–1050, 1995.

- Increased postprandial lipemia (slow clearance of fat from the blood)
- Smaller, denser LDL cholesterol particles
- Excess fibrinogen
- Excess PAI-1
- Hypertension

Add to these the lifestyle habits that worsen Syndrome X:

- Obesity
- Lack of physical activity
- The wrong diet
- Cigarette smoking

And throw in the independent risk factor that affects us all, whether or not we have Syndrome X:

- Higher than normal LDL cholesterol

Taken all together, it's clear that Syndrome X is more than a disease with a single cause and a clear-cut progression. It is a large cluster of changes in metabolism, the blood and the blood pressure. Although being insulin resistant does not, by itself, mean that you will develop Syndrome X, it is clear that the combination of insulin resistance and compensatory hyperinsulinemia increases your risk of developing the disease. It's possible you may have just a few manifestations, or you may have all—a lot depends on your genetic makeup and your health and lifestyle habits.

THE JOURNEY FROM

INSULIN RESISTANCE

TO SYNDROME X

THE "BIRTH" OF SYNDROME X was a complex affair, a long process of piecing together theories and findings that seemed to fly in the face of the best medical knowledge.

I first described the cluster of heart attack risk factors associated with insulin resistance, and suggested the name Syndrome X, back in 1988, in New Orleans. There to receive the American Diabetes Association's Banting Medal for Scientific Research, the highest research award given by that association, I described the sequence of research findings that led to our understanding of the syndrome.

The story begins with a set of observations made by myself and other researchers. These apparently unrelated items formed the foundation for the research that eventually led to Syndrome X.

1. *Triglycerides (blood fats) contribute to heart attacks.* Until the 1950s, cholesterol was considered the primary culprit in heart disease. But Yale University scientists challenged this notion late in that decade, when they showed that patients who had suffered heart attacks were more likely to have high triglycerides than they were to have elevated cholesterol levels. Despite the Yale University researchers' very persuasive evidence, the medical

community was not ready to accept this new idea. But the data intrigued me; I wanted to know more.

2. *Blood fat levels respond differently in different people.* When researchers first identified elevated blood triglycerides as a risk factor for heart attack, it was not easy to measure triglyceride levels, and doctors didn't really know what made them rise and fall. Then researchers at the Rockefeller Institute published a series of research papers showing that different diets had different effects on triglyceride levels. In the vast majority of those with high blood fats ("essential lipemia"), levels rose when they ate a high-carbohydrate diet, and fell when they consumed a high-fat diet. But in a small minority, the results were reversed. This seemed odd. Why would high blood triglycerides be induced by carbohydrates in most people, and by fat in the remaining few? Why wouldn't more dietary fat always make the level rise, and less fat always make it fall?

3. *Both glucose levels and insulin levels can be high in those with type 2 diabetes.* In the late 1950s, two investigators from the Bronx Veterans Administration Hospital astonished the medical community when they showed that patients with type 2 diabetes could have elevated glucose levels despite also having higher insulin levels. You would think that high insulin levels would have prevented type 2 diabetes, that the "extra" insulin would push the glucose into their cells. But their blood sugars remained high. The results seemed to suggest that type 2 diabetics must not respond normally to their insulin; otherwise, why would both their insulin and glucose levels be high? .

4. *Heart attacks are more common in those with disturbed glucose tolerance than in normal people.*

Intrigued by these observations, I theorized that people whose glucose tolerances were not absolutely normal were at greater risk for heart disease, just like those with type 2 diabetes. I designed my first study at Stanford University School of Medicine to test this out. We enlisted and divided our volunteers into two groups. Neither group included diabetics, but the members of one group had suffered heart attacks. Those in the other group, the control group, had not. Everybody was given a glucose tolerance test, and the results were interesting. The "previous heart attack" group had high blood sugar levels during the glucose tolerance tests. And, like those in the Yale studies, they also had high triglyceride levels.

What did this mean? Was there a relationship between blood triglyceride levels, glucose, insulin, the way blood fats respond to food, type 2 diabetes and heart attack? How did it all fit together? Advances in medical science often come about when someone tries to explain why certain things happen by developing a new hypothesis that links together what seem to be unrelated pieces of information. That's exactly what happened with Syndrome X. My research group took the first of a series of steps leading to Syndrome X by proposing a new hypothesis that provided one explanation for the four observations. Our premise was based on a series of new ideas:

- The ability of insulin to stimulate the uptake of glucose by muscle cells must vary considerably from person to person.
- Some insulin-resistant people can secrete enough insulin to overcome their resistance and prevent type 2 diabetes.
- The higher insulin levels resulting from insulin resistance cause the liver to increase its production of triglyceride-rich VLDL and release it into the bloodstream.
- The increased VLDL in the bloodstream raises triglyceride concentration (blood fats) and increases the risk of coronary heart disease.
- The more carbohydrate an insulin-resistant person eats, the more insulin the pancreas must secrete to prevent the blood glucose from climbing too high. The higher the blood insulin levels, the greater the production of VLDL, and the more the triglyceride levels will rise.

If all this was true, it would begin to define and explain the link between blood fat, glucose, insulin, type 2 diabetes and heart attack. But could we prove our hypothesis? We approached the complex hypothesis step by step.

We began by testing the crucial arm of our theory: are there more triglycerides in the blood because the liver has made more? We developed a reliable new testing method, and were exhilarated to discover that there is an extremely close relationship between the amount of triglyceride-rich VLDL secreted by the liver and the amount of triglyceride in the blood. The first step was successfully completed.

Having shown that blood levels of triglyceride rose when the liver put out more VLDL, we now wanted to link elevated insulin levels with higher triglyceride concentrations. By measuring plasma insulin and triglyceride concentrations throughout the day in response to meals, we clearly showed that the higher the level of insulin in the blood, the more triglyceride-rich VLDL the body produces and the higher the triglyceride levels.

Next, we needed to prove that high insulin levels in people with normal amounts of blood glucose really meant that they were insulin resistant. We thought this was so, but belief is one thing, scientific proof quite another. To proceed, we had to devise a method of measuring insulin resistance. By 1968, we had done so and tested it out by comparing normal individuals to patients with type 2 diabetes. The results of our initial studies provided the first quantitative evidence of the severity of insulin resistance in patients with type 2 diabetes. We then applied the same test to nondiabetics, our excitement growing as we confirmed that insulin resistance varies considerably in nondiabetic people, and the more insulin resistant a nondiabetic was, the higher the plasma insulin concentration. Not only did insulin rise with insulin resistance, but as the insulin levels went up, so did the triglyceride concentration.

So far, so good. Everything we had proposed bore out under scientific scrutiny. We showed that increased insulin resistance led to higher levels of insulin in the blood, which prompted the liver to synthesize and release more VLDL into the blood. This, in turn, caused blood triglyceride levels to rise. We had just one more experiment to conduct, the ultimate test: what happens when people eat more carbohydrate? Does that cause insulin levels to rise in the insulin-resistant? The results were just what we anticipated. The more carbohydrates eaten, the more the insulin levels increased, the more triglyceride-rich VLDL the liver produced and secreted, and the higher the plasma triglyceride concentrations. In other words, the more insulin resistant one was, the greater the negative impact of a high-carbohydrate diet.

We had scientifically proven every aspect of our hypothesis. The groundwork for Syndrome X had been laid, but a lot of hard work remained ahead.

Complicating and Completing the Equation

While our team was performing the experiments that formed the basis of Syndrome X, other researchers were gathering more evidence. For example, it became apparent that you could have a heart attack even if your LDL cholesterol was within the normal range. We also learned that the HDL cholesterol figured into the equation: several studies clearly showed that risk of heart attack was at least as great in people with low HDL cholesterols as it was in those with elevated LDL cholesterols. (This new information led to the distinction between "good" HDL cholesterol and "bad" LDL cholesterol.) Further increasing heart attack risk was the fact that a low HDL often came in conjunction with high blood triglyceride levels.

Once this correlation was clear, we hypothesized that people with low HDL cholesterols were most likely insulin resistant, and had high insulin levels. Our experiments confirmed that this was true. Low HDL cholesterol joined high triglyceride levels in the Syndrome X cluster.

High blood pressure became linked to Syndrome X when we began to wonder why many people with hypertension continued to have heart attacks, despite the availability of good medicines to lower blood pressure. Could it be because many people with hypertension had manifestations of Syndrome X, which were unaffected by the blood pressure medications? It was relatively easy to test this out, and we now know that approximately 50 percent of patients with high blood pressure are insulin resistant and have high blood insulin levels, as well as other manifestations of the syndrome. Our later research showed that people with Syndrome X who also have high blood pressure are at the greatest risk of heart attack.

Linking low HDL cholesterol and elevated blood pressure to Syndrome X brought us full circle, back to my presentation at the American Diabetes Association meeting in 1988. There, I defined Syndrome X as a cluster of abnormalities associated with insulin resistance. When full-blown, I explained, it induced slightly higher-than-normal glucose levels, compensatory hyperinsulinemia, elevated blood triglycerides, low HDL cholesterol and high blood pressure. Since then, research has prompted us to add a few more components to the Syndrome X cluster, including smaller, denser LDL particles, slow clearing of blood fats after meals (exaggerated postprandial lipemia) and poor ability to break up blood clots (dysfibrinolysis). The list of Syndrome X manifestations has grown, and I suspect that in time more will be added.

FROM SYNDROME X TO HEART ATTACK

How does insulin resistance trigger the metabolic changes that comprise the syndrome and lead to heart attack? How does it cause:

- glucose intolerance
- excess blood fat (hypertriglyceridemia)
- slow clearing of blood fats after meals (exaggerated postprandial lipemia)
- low HDL cholesterol levels
- small, dense LDL particles
- disturbances in blood clotting (dysfibrinolysis)
- elevated blood pressure (hypertension)

In Chapter 3 we saw how these manifestations of the syndrome can trigger a heart attack. Now let's see what sets them in motion.

Glucose Intolerance. The body's ability to handle glucose is affected by genetics and lifestyle. The more insulin resistant you are, the more difficult it is for your pancreas to secrete enough insulin to keep your blood sugar in the desired range. Even if you're not diabetic, your blood glucose concentrations are a little higher throughout the day, and don't bounce down to baseline as quickly. For example, blood glucose in an insulin-sensitive individual with absolutely normal glucose tolerance will rise no higher than 140 mg/dl after a meal, and drop back down to normal within two hours. But in an insulin-resistant person with glucose intolerance, blood sugar might go as high as 160 mg/dl after a meal, and take perhaps thirty minutes longer to return to the pre-meal level. This isn't bad enough to qualify as type 2 diabetes, but it's not healthy. Approximately 25 percent of the nondiabetic population with the highest glucose levels are at increased risk for heart attack.

Too Much Blood Fat (Hypertriglyceridemia). Triglycerides are made in the liver. The most important factors that determine how much triglyceride your liver makes are the day-long levels of insulin and fatty acids in your blood. Simply put, fatty acids are raw materials for the liver's triglyceride assembly line, and excess insulin makes that line go faster. Insulin resistance in adipose (fat) cells causes them to release more of the fatty acids they store, which makes more raw material available to the liver. Meanwhile, insulin resistance in muscle cells leads to excess insulin in the blood, which spurs the liver's production of triglyceride. The liver assembles and releases larger amounts of the triglyceride-rich VLDL, and blood triglyceride levels rise.

Slowed Clearing of Blood Fats After Meals (Exaggerated Postprandial Lipemia). Unfortunately, we humans have a limited ability to clear fat from the blood; we process only so much at a time. Syndrome X sufferers are even slower because they begin the day with higher triglyceride levels and, as recently released studies have shown, their insulin resistance further reduces their ability to clear away blood fat after meals. Unfortunately, as several recent publications have emphasized, a postprandial increase in triglyceride-rich lipoproteins is a risk factor for heart attack. Indeed, there is good evidence that the remnant particles formed as triglyceride is removed from the chylomicrons and VLDL are particularly good at spurring on the atherosclerotic process.

Low HDL "Good" Cholesterol. When insulin and triglyceride concentrations rise, HDL cholesterol falls. This is exactly what happens with Syndrome X. As you remember from Chapter 3, an enzyme called CETP plays a vital role in transferring cholesterol from HDL to VLDL, in exchange for triglyceride. The unfortunate result is more VLDL cholesterol and less protective HDL cholesterol. The more VLDL in the bloodstream, the more opportunity for this dangerous exchange to occur—and people with Syndrome X have more VLDL. In addition, experiments from several research laboratories, including mine at Stanford, have shown that the more insulin resistant and hyperinsulinemic you are, the faster the protein in HDL is removed from the circulation and the lower your HDL cholesterol.

Small, Dense LDL Particles. We've long been puzzled by the fact that many heart attack victims do not have elevated LDL cholesterol, even though it is a major risk factor. Examining this paradox, we learned that heart attack victims were about as likely to have high triglycerides and low HDL cholesterols as they were to have elevated LDL. Furthermore, we found that the LDL particle itself was different—it was smaller and denser. Smaller and denser LDL particles, along with a high triglyceride level and low HDL cholesterol, are predictive of heart attack.

The appearance of smaller and denser LDL particles was closely associated with the abnormal lipoprotein metabolism characterizing Syndrome X. Thus, we were not surprised when my research group showed that insulin resistance and hyperinsulinemia were associated with these smaller, denser LDL particles. We're not quite sure why smaller, denser LDL increases the risk of heart attack so much. Preliminary evidence suggests it is because these particles can be more easily oxidized, making them more likely to damage artery linings. In support of this hypothesis, my team has recently published research data linking together insulin resistance, hyperinsulinemia and the ease with which LDL particles can be oxidized.

Disturbances in Blood Clotting (Dysfibrinolysis).PAI-1 plays a major role in regulating the body's making and breaking up of clots. The higher the PAI-1 levels, the less the body is able to dissolve clots. Elevated PAI-1 is now a well-recognized risk factor for heart attack.

Earlier studies found that a high PAI-1 level went hand in hand with elevated triglycerides and low HDL cholesterol. It wasn't long before several studies were published showing that a high PAI-1 was part of Syndrome X. Perhaps the most persuasive of these is a report from Europe of a large, collaborative study of 1,500 patients with angina pectoris. In these individuals with clear-cut coronary heart disease, there was a very close association between increases in PAI-1 and insulin levels and all of the other manifestations of Syndrome X.

Both insulin and triglyceride act on certain cells to increase the synthesis and secretion of PAI-1 into the bloodstream, although we don't yet know whether insulin or triglyceride plays the greater role. However, since increases in both insulin and triglyceride characterize Syndrome X, it should not be surprising that a high blood level of PAI-1 is part of the cluster.

The story with fibrinogen is even less clear. At present, the best explanation is that changes in the blood vessel walls that occur in individuals with Syndrome X lead to increased production of fibrinogen.

High Blood Pressure (Hypertension). We aren't absolutely sure why insulin resistance leads to hypertension, although studies suggest two possible, related explanations. First, there is good evidence suggesting that hyperinsulinemia encourages the kidneys to retain salt—and water along with it. More salt and water in the body means a greater volume of blood coursing through the blood vessels, and pressure goes up. Insulin-resistant patients with hypertension are usually salt sensitive; their blood pressures go up when they consume more salt. Generally speaking, the higher the insulin level, the greater the risk of retaining salt.

The second theory has to do with the blood vessels. Excess insulin acts on the sympathetic nervous system which, in turn, causes the arteries to decrease in diameter. It also increases the activity of hormones, called catecholamines, that decrease a blood vessel's diameter. Acting through both the nervous system and catecholamines, excess insulin narrows arteries, making it harder for blood to flow through and pushing up blood pressure. To make matters worse, the increase in sympathetic nervous system activity increases salt retention by the kidney. We don't know which is worse for your blood pressure—the effects of hyperinsulinemia on the kidney or on the sympathetic nervous system. But we do know that high blood pressure commonly develops in the insulin resistant, that it is part of Syndrome X and that it increases the risk of heart attack.

These are the problems wrought by Syndrome X. But what are its causes?

WHAT CAUSES SYNDROME X?

With some diseases, such as strep throat, the cause and effect are obvious. One of the various forms of streptococcal bacteria gets into your body, takes up residence in your throat and you develop a sore throat, fever, headache and/or other symptoms. Within about two weeks your immune system defeats the offending bacteria, or perhaps antibiotics do the trick, and all is well.

But Syndrome X is not a single disease with a single cause. It's not triggered by one germ, an unhealthful diet, an injury or a solitary genetic abnormality. Instead, it's the result of a series of metabolic changes that tend to occur in people who are insulin resistant. As time passes, a cluster of these alterations may develop, resulting in a full-blown case of Syndrome X.

In order to understand why some people are more likely than others to develop the manifestations of Syndrome X, we must first see why some are insulin resistant while others are insulin sensitive. And it's not even a simple matter of insulin resistance versus insulin sensitivity, for the ability of insulin to do its job can vary tenfold in apparently healthy people.

Genes and Insulin Resistance

Insulin instructs certain cells to "open the door" to glucose, but there's more to it than insulin issuing a simple command to "open sesame." Rather, it's a multistep process that begins when insulin binds to specific receptors on the outside of a cell. Acting through the "insulin signal transduction mechanism," the cell responds by generating a series of signals instructing carrier proteins called GLUT 4 transporters to move to the cell surface. These GLUT 4 transporters hurry to the cell membranes and help glucose move from your bloodstream into your cells.

This complex process is guided by many genes; an abnormality in one or more of these genes might be responsible for insulin resistance. As yet, we don't know which specific genes might be at fault, or if the abnormality occurs in the same way in all people. A complex set of genetic errors is most likely to blame, and the makeup of this set probably varies from person to person.

Are Genes Really to Blame?

If we don't know which genetic errors are responsible for insulin resistance, how can we conclude that genes play any role at all? The truth is, we can't be 100 percent sure. But evidence gathered from three separate lines of research points an accusatory finger directly at our genes.

The first line of evidence emerged from measuring insulin action and related lifestyle variables in healthy individuals. (See box below.) Working with researchers in Phoenix, Arizona, we measured insulin resistance in healthy volunteers of European and Native American ancestry living in either the San Francisco Bay area or outside of Phoenix, Arizona. The results showed that approximately 50 percent of the variability in insulin action from person to person can be attributed to differences in lifestyle. By default, we can conclude that the remaining 50 percent variability is due to genetic differences.

Half and Half—and Half Again

In an early study exploring the relationship between genes and insulin resistance, we enlisted ninety healthy nondiabetic volunteers. Fifty-five were Pima Indians, the remaining thirty-five were Caucasians living in California. All males, they ranged in age from eighteen to seventy-five. The results were published in *The American Journal of Physiology* in 1985.*

In our laboratories at Stanford University and Phoenix, Arizona, we took these measurements:

- an estimate of how fat (obese) the volunteers were
- their degree of physical fitness as determined by their performance while walking on a treadmill
- the effectiveness of their insulin in increasing the rate at which their bodies utilized glucose

Then we used statistical techniques to determine the degree to which differences in their degree of fatness and fitness contributed to the variability of their insulin action. The answer was half and half, then half of that. More specifically, half of the variability of insulin action was due to lifestyle, the other half presumably to our genes. Of the 50 percent attributed to lifestyle, half was due to fitness, half to obesity.

* C. Bogardus et al. "Relationship between degree of obesity and in vivo insulin action in the man." *The American Journal of Physiology* (1985) 248:E286–E291.

The second line of evidence came from studying families. For these investigations, insulin resistance was measured in each of several members of many families. Members of the same family, of course, have very similar genetic backgrounds. This study found that the ability of insulin to stimulate cells to take in glucose was much more alike within families than it was from family to family. In other words, if one person was insulin resistant, his or her siblings were statistically more likely to be insulin resistant. This clustering of insulin action within families supported the argument that genes play a major role in insulin resistance.

Brothers, Sisters and Insulin Resistance

Forty-five Pima Indian families, ranging in size from two to six, participated in a study* conducted in Phoenix, Arizona. The degree of insulin resistance was determined by measuring how effective insulin was in stimulating the body's use of glucose. Statistical methods were then used to see if the similarity of the measure was more alike in family members than it was when comparing individuals in different families. The answer was straightforward: your degree of insulin resistance is much more like your sibling's than your best friend's.

* S. Lillioja, D. M. Mott, J. K. Zawadzki, et al. "In vivo insulin action is a familial characteristic in non-diabetic Pima Indians." *Diabetes* (1987) 36:1329–1335.

The third line of evidence sprang from population studies looking at insulin resistance in healthy volunteers from different ethnic groups. The results of many studies have shown that insulin resistance is greater in American Indians, South Asian Indians, Japanese-Americans, African-Americans, Mexican-Americans, Australian Aboriginals and various Pacific Island populations, compared to those of European ancestry. (It's theoretically possible that some groups are more insulin resistant than others primarily because of lifestyle habits rather than genetics, but several studies took all known factors into account.)

The results of these studies of individuals, families and large population groups all suggested that genes play a major role in the development of insulin resistance, and that people of non-European ancestry are more likely to have the offending genes. Assuming that's true, non-Europeans should be more likely to develop Syndrome X and suffer from heart attacks. Here lay an opportunity to test the theory that genes are responsible by picking out a group with "insulin resistant genes" and determining whether or not its members had more heart disease.

That's just what researchers did. The best documented case involves South Asian Indians living in the United Kingdom. Although they ate little fat and had lower cholesterol levels then their European neighbors down the street, they suffered from a 50 percent greater incidence of type 2 diabetes and heart attacks. Clearly, genes played a major role in the development of insulin resistance and Syndrome X in these South Asian Indians.

Lifestyle and Insulin Resistance

If genes are 50 percent responsible for the development of Syndrome X, lifestyle habits must account for the other half. Let's look again at insulin-resistant South Asian Indians to demonstrate the role of lifestyle. Researchers have found that South Asian Indians living in India are less likely to suffer heart attacks than South Asian Indians living in Europe or the United States. Why? The differences between members of the same ethnic group living in different countries cannot be due to genetic factors, for they share the same genes. They have to be related to differences in lifestyle.

The fact that lifestyle is "half to blame" for the variability in insulin action from person to person—and, therefore, the development of Syndrome X—can be good or bad news, depending on your perspective. The good news is that you're in control, you can defeat the disease by making lifestyle changes. The bad news is that you're in control, and changing your lifestyle can be difficult—you can't just rely on a pill or a simple surgery to solve the problem. It's tough to undo a lifetime's worth of habits and preferences. But it's well worth the effort.

Several aspects of lifestyle affect Syndrome X: body weight, level of physical activity, smoking, alcohol consumption and diet. The first two, body weight and physical activity, are powerful tools for controlling Syndrome X, and are usually more effective than medications. (We'll look at the effects of smoking and drinking on Syndrome X in Chapter 9, and discuss the relationship between body weight, physical activity and Syndrome X in detail in Chapters 7 and 8. For now, just a few words on obesity and physical activity.)

Obesity worsens all the manifestations of Syndrome X. The primary link between being overweight and an increased risk of a Syndrome X–induced heart attack is straightforward:

- The more obese you are, the more insulin resistant you will be.
- The more insulin resistant you become, the more insulin you secrete.
- The higher your insulin levels, the more likely you are to develop the manifestations of Syndrome X and the greater your odds of developing heart disease.

In the simplest sense, obesity results from an imbalance between energy intake (calories in) and energy output (calories burned during physical activity plus the calories burned every day just to stay alive). It's like a bank account: if you deposit more money (calories) than you withdraw (physical activity), your bank account (body weight) grows. If you withdraw more calories than you put in, your balance falls. It doesn't matter what kind of money (dollars, lira, pounds) you put into your bank account, or how that money is withdrawn (cash, check, cashier's check). Neither does it matter what "kind" of calories (protein, fat, carbohydrate) you eat or how you burn them off (running, bicycling, strolling, dancing). Calories in minus calories out is the only equation that counts when it comes to losing weight.

When it comes to insulin resistance/sensitivity, however, obesity is not an either-or situation of being either obese and insulin resistant, or slim and insulin sensitive. Not every obese person is insulin resistant, and not all slender people are insulin sensitive. Obesity is but one of the factors interacting with your genes to determine the ability of your tissues to react to insulin. If you are genetically more insulin sensitive to begin with, weight gain will have a less pronounced effect on your risk of developing Syndrome X. Unfortunately, the opposite is equally true. If you are genetically more insulin resistant, becoming obese can create far more damaging effects.

When many early experiments showed that obesity made insulin action worse, we took it for granted that the extra pounds alone were to blame. Today we know that it's not just those excess pounds that increase insulin resistance, but what tends to go along with them. Obese people are often physically inactive, and variations in physical activity are as powerful as the degree of obesity when it comes to modifying the ability of insulin to stimulate glucose uptake.

In other words, obesity is usually a double-whammy against insulin sensitivity. Even if someone has inherited insulin-sensitive genes, the combination of obesity and physical inactivity can be overwhelming. We cannot change our genes, but we can modify our lifestyles. No matter what your genetic background, you can take major steps toward decreasing the ravages of Syndrome X (or keeping it entirely at bay) by staying active. Doing so helps directly by increasing insulin sensitivity, and indirectly by helping you shed the excess pounds that interfere with insulin's action.

The Simple

Solution

THE SIX-STEP

SYNDROME X PROGRAM

LIKE A LOT OF people, sixty-five-year-old Dorothy was puzzled, frightened and angry when she found out that the "best" medical advice was actually detrimental to her health. As she tells it:

> Six years ago, at my annual checkup, my doctor told me that my blood pressure had been creeping up bit by bit for years, and now it was too high. She said that was normal for someone my age—I was fifty-nine years old then. That surprised me, because even though I tired easily, I didn't feel bad. But she said most people have no symptoms of high blood pressure until it gets sky high, and she insisted that we do something about it right away, before it got out of control.
>
> That made sense, so I began to take the diuretic she prescribed every day, which lowered my blood pressure some, but not enough. So my doctor gave me another medicine that was supposed to lower it even further. Together, the two medicines finally got my pressure down to an acceptable level.
>
> The next year was great. I felt good, I had enough energy to do a lot of work in the garden and I even took a little trip to the Caribbean. But one afternoon, while I was planting petunias, I felt this squeezing kind of pain in my chest. I sat there for, I don't know, ten or fifteen minutes wait-

ing for it to go away. But it didn't. Then my jaw and my left arm started to hurt, and I was having trouble breathing. I thought maybe I should go inside, so I stood up—and boy, did that make me dizzy! So I half-walked over to my next-door neighbor's house and asked her to take me to the emergency room.

All the way to the hospital I told myself, over and over, that this couldn't be a heart attack. It couldn't possibly be, because I took my medicines every single day, and my blood pressure was under good control. But when I got to the emergency room, the doctors there ordered all kinds of tests. Then they put me in the coronary care unit and left me there in bed, hooked up to a heart monitor.

The next day, another doctor came in and told me I'd had a small heart attack! I said that couldn't be, because the medicines had controlled my blood pressure. He just shrugged his shoulders and said that lowering blood pressure helped decrease the risk of heart attack, but it was not a guarantee.

I was really scared! Would I have another heart attack? What good was taking the two medicines if they couldn't prevent this from happening? I was also angry with my doctor—really angry—because I thought she'd told me that the blood pressure medicines would take away my risk of having a heart attack.

Fortunately, I recovered quickly from the heart attack. I thought it would be a good idea to get a second opinion about my condition, so I saw Dr. Gerald Reaven at Stanford. He told me that my case was not unusual. "People with high blood pressure often have other risk factors for heart disease," he explained, "different ones that can be just as dangerous." Dr. Reaven ordered some blood tests. When I returned for my second appointment, he said: "You have Syndrome X, a cluster of metabolic abnormalities that increase the risk of heart disease. Your glucose is high, but not high enough to indicate diabetes. Your triglycerides are high and your HDL cholesterol is only 36, which is too low. You should also lose some weight, perhaps ten or fifteen pounds. If you do this, you'll have a much smaller risk of suffering a heart attack, whether induced by Syndrome X or other causes. I'm going to put you on a program to overcome Syndrome X. The special diet and the exercise programs will help you lose weight while controlling your blood sugar. Even though the diet lets you eat more fat than most diets, it's the 'good' fat that helps keep your heart healthy."

Five years have gone by since then, and I haven't had another heart attack. I feel great, I've lost thirteen pounds and I've got more energy than ever! And the doctor was right—following the diet and losing weight improved all my numbers. My triglycerides and my blood sugar both went down, and my HDL went up. I've pretty much stopped worry-ing about having another heart attack. Instead, I'm planning on sticking around for a long time—long enough to watch my grandkids and my great-grandkids grow up!

Dorothy made wonderful progress on our Six-Step Syndrome X Program. The weight loss diet she was given, together with increased exercise, helped her lose most of the excess weight she'd been carry-ing around. She had never smoked, so that wasn't a problem, and she was still able to enjoy one cocktail per day, since there is no evidence that a moderate alcohol intake increases the risk of Syndrome X and heart attack. The combination of her lifestyle changes and her blood pressure medication helped Dorothy reduce her Syndrome X risk fac-tors considerably; in fact, the risk factors had totally disappeared within six months. Dorothy has had little difficulty maintaining her new, healthier and more vigorous lifestyle, and today has more en-ergy than ever.

A COMPLEX PROBLEM BEYOND JUST CHOLESTEROL

Millions of Americans are concerned about their cholesterol levels, and rightly so, for many of us are well into the danger zone. To com-bat this problem, we now have over three hundred medicines to help us control cholesterol levels and otherwise keep our hearts healthy. Descriptions of these drugs fill more than four hundred pages of the *Physician's Desk Reference*, the "bible" of medications. But looking at the world through cholesterol-colored glasses can prevent you from seeing other potential dangers to heart health, such as the risk factors associated with Syndrome X. You can have a healthy LDL cholesterol and still be hit with a heart attack induced by the syndrome.

If you have insulin resistance and compensatory hyperinsuline-mia, simply lowering your total cholesterol probably won't prevent a heart attack. Exercising won't shield you completely, and neither will eating a low-fat, low-cholesterol diet. These are all helpful steps, but they only nibble away at the "edges" of the problem, never getting to the core of Syndrome X risk factors.

Elevated total cholesterol, which many people are concerned about, doesn't even appear on the Syndrome X risk factor list. Neither does a high LDL cholesterol. Having too much LDL "bad" cholesterol increases the risk of suffering a heart attack for everyone, but is not a part of Syndrome X. That's not to say, of course, that you should ignore your total cholesterol or LDL "bad" cholesterol levels. An elevated LDL cholesterol level, cigarette smoking and obesity are health problems for everyone, whether Syndrome X is present or not. But remember that if you have Syndrome X, you have more to consider.

You can see how complex the Syndrome X equation is, how many different elements must be considered, when its risk factors are listed according to the body system affected:

Insulin/glucose abnormalities
- Impaired glucose tolerance
- High insulin levels (hyperinsulinemia)

Cholesterol
- Low HDL "good" cholesterol
- Smaller, more dense LDL particles

Blood fat
- Elevated triglycerides (blood fats)
- Slow clearance of fat from the blood (exaggerated postprandial lipemia)

Blood clotting
- Increased propensity of the blood to form clots
- Decreased ability to dispose of blood clots

Circulatory
- Elevated blood pressure

Systemic/lifestyle
- Obesity
- Lack of physical activity
- The wrong diet
- Cigarette smoking

All of these problems must be dealt with simultaneously if you are to conquer Syndrome X.

A SIMPLE PLAN CURES A COMPLEX PROBLEM

Here's the Six-Step Syndrome X Program. Based on good science, backed by solid documentation and many published studies, it will work on all the syndrome's risk factors at once (and significantly reduce the "bad" LDL cholesterol):

Step 1. Diagnosis
Step 2. The Syndrome X Diet™
Step 3. Weight Loss
Step 4. Physical Activity
Step 5. Healthy Lifestyle Habits
Step 6. Medical Intervention (if necessary)

Let's take a closer look at these steps.

Step 1. Diagnosis

It's easy to discover whether or not you have Syndrome X. There are no exotic or expensive tests, you don't have to go to a major hospital or research center. The necessary tests are simple and commonplace; they're already performed thousands of times a day all across the country. Unfortunately, not all physicians know which tests to perform and how to interpret the results. Many doctors wouldn't notice if you have Syndrome X because they don't know what to look for.

Here are five of the most easily identifiable predictors of Syndrome X. Ask your doctor to give you these tests:

- *Glucose tolerance test.* Eat no food (although you may drink water) after eight o'clock the night before your test; then go to your doctor and have blood drawn before you eat the next morning. Have your glucose measured in the fasting state (before eating in the morning), then again one and two hours after drinking 75 grams of glucose.
- *Triglycerides (blood fats).* Have your blood fat levels measured with the first, fasting blood taken for the glucose tolerance test.
- *HDL cholesterol.* Have your HDL cholesterol level measured with the first, fasting blood taken for the glucose tolerance test.
- *Blood pressure.* Have your doctor check to see if your blood pressure is elevated (above 145/90).
- *Weight check.* Ask your doctor if you are overweight. If you are overweight, ask your doctor by how many pounds.

Working with your doctor, use your test results and the scoring system below to assess your risk of heart attack due to Syndrome X. If your doctor does not know about Syndrome X or hesitates to share your test results, insist on getting "the numbers" from him or her and evaluate your risk of heart attack yourself.

Self-Assessment for Risk of Syndrome X

If Your	Give Yourself
■ Fasting glucose level is greater than 110, or your glucose at two hours into the Glucose Tolerance Test is greater than 140	3 points
■ Fasting triglyceride level is greater than 200	3 points
■ Fasting HDL-cholesterol level is lower than 35	3 points
■ Blood pressure is greater than 145/90	3 points
■ Weight check reveals you are more than 15 pounds overweight	1 point
■ Family has a history of heart disease, high blood pressure (hypertension) or diabetes	1 point
■ Lifestyle is characterized by physical inactivity in both work and leisure hours	½ point
TOTAL SCORE _____ points	

If You Scored	Your Risk of Heart Attack Triggered by Syndrome X Is:
0–4 points	Low
5–8 points	Moderate
9–12 points	High
13 points or more	Very high

The higher your total score, the greater your potential risk of heart attack due to Syndrome X. But you may be at risk even if your score seems low. *If you have these risk factors, especially any of the first four, see a physician familiar with the syndrome.*

If you scored moderate to high, don't despair. Start the Six-Step Program and begin working to reduce your risk of heart attack due to Syndrome X.

We've been discussing the risk of developing a heart attack triggered by Syndrome X, but don't forget that you can have an attack for other reasons. Even if you don't have the syndrome, be sure to have your LDL and other heart attack risk factors carefully monitored by your physician.

Isn't Something Missing from the Test?

Why isn't a measure of the insulin concentration in the blood included in the Self-Assessment for Risk of Syndrome X? After all, isn't the problem caused by insulin resistance and the resulting "extra" insulin in the bloodstream?

Simply put, knowing how much insulin is in the blood at a given time is not that helpful, not for our purposes. The results of insulin tests vary depending on which laboratory conducts the analysis, and there is no universally agreed upon range of "normal" insulin levels. Furthermore, it's possible to be insulin resistant and have high insulin concentrations, but not have Syndrome X. This is not likely, but it is a consideration. That's why the diagnosis is based on the presence of the syndrome's manifestations, such as elevated triglyceride and low HDL cholesterol levels, not the "raw" amount of insulin in the blood.

Step 2. The Syndrome X Diet™

Odds are your physician and health-oriented friends have been telling you to cut back on fat and eat more carbohydrates. That may be good advice for some of us, but it's not the best advice for those with Syndrome X.

You need carefully balanced proportions of carbohydrate, protein and fat. Some popular diets are fairly good for keeping insulin under control but, ironically, they can increase your risk of heart disease by raising your LDL "bad" cholesterol levels. And there are diets that help lower your LDL, but may send your insulin soaring if you have the syndrome. The Syndrome X Diet is the only approach that keeps insulin under control and pushes LDL cholesterol down.

Drawing 45 percent of its calories from carbohydrate, 40 percent from fat and 15 percent from protein, the Syndrome X Diet is the foundation of the program. But it's a controversial approach, flying in the face of accepted wisdom offered by venerable health institutions such as the American Heart Association, the American Diabetes Association and the National Cholesterol Education Program. These and other groups insist that low-fat diets are best for everyone—but they aren't!

Don't let that shake your resolve. Most well-meaning physicians, dietitians and organizations are simply unaware of Syndrome X and its ramifications. Their dietary advice doesn't take the syndrome into account. Their advice to all Americans to replace fat with carbohydrate is fine for many of us, but if you have Syndrome X, too much carbohydrate can lead to trouble.

Step 3. Weight Loss

The closer you are to your ideal body weight the better, for the insulin resistance that lies at the heart of Syndrome X grows worse as excess pounds pile on. The more obese you become, the more insulin your body must produce to keep glucose under control, and the greater the damage caused by Syndrome X.

Slimming down helps lower insulin levels by making your insulin more effective, thus reducing the risk from all the Syndrome X risk factors. And it's beneficial to remain slim even if you don't have Syndrome X, for obesity is a universal risk factor for heart disease.

Most people can shed excess pounds with judicious eating and regular exercise. The weight loss menus that you'll find in Chapters 15 and 16 are easy to prepare, easy to follow and easy to stick with. You'll be able to enjoy delicious meals without suffering.

Step 4. Physical Activity

Obesity and lack of physical activity don't cause Syndrome X, but they do make it worse. That's why exercise is one of the best "medicines" for people with the syndrome. It attacks the fundamental problem by lowering insulin and blood triglyceride levels, and raising the HDL cholesterol. Although we have not yet conducted the studies to prove this is so, exercise should theoretically also make the LDL particles larger and less dense, speed the clearance of blood fats from your system and decrease the likelihood that you'll develop unnecessary blood clots.

Fortunately, you needn't run marathons to benefit. In Chapter 8 we'll look at ways to make exercise a regular part of your day, every day, even if you have difficulty simply standing up for long.

Step 5. Healthy Lifestyle Habits

Alcohol and cigarettes are part of many people's lives. While moderate consumption of alcohol does not pose a danger for those with Syndrome X, there is absolutely no doubt that smoking does. The results of studies conducted in our laboratories demonstrated that smokers are significantly more insulin resistant and have higher insulin levels than do nonsmokers, and confirmed that they have higher blood triglyceride and lower HDL cholesterol levels. In short, smoking cigarettes increases your likelihood of developing Syndrome X, and can give the syndrome extra "punch." And there are, of course, many other reasons to stop smoking.

Step 6. Medical Intervention (If Necessary)

Although the first five points of the program will suffice for many people, some will require medicines to keep their triglyceride, blood pressure and LDL cholesterol levels under control.

If you do need medicine, carefully consider the drugs you take, for their side effects can make things worse. For example, some medicines used to lower blood pressure can push the LDL and triglyceride levels up, while lowering the HDL. Chapter 10 looks at medicines that can complement your lifestyle changes.

ONE PROGRAM, MANY APPROACHES

Syndrome X is a complicated disorder, making it impossible to come up with a magical, "one size fits all" program to keep it under control. Nonetheless, it will be relatively easy for you to find your own best solution. Your Syndrome X strategy will be based primarily on your laboratory test results.

Which strategy you use depends on how many aspects of Syndrome X you have, and how severe they are. Some people develop all the aspects of the syndrome, others only one or two. In some people the aspects are strong, in others they're mild to middling. But even if you are only standing on the precipice of Syndrome X, taking action now will greatly increase the odds that you'll avoid heart disease.

THE SYNDROME X DIET™

CAROLYN FRY, A FIFTY-FOUR-YEAR-OLD Silicon Valley computer programmer, was a veteran dieter. She had tried every popular diet, from the Atkins diet to The Zone. She had lost a few pounds on each, but invariably gained it all back within six months. Her weight, as a result, had seesawed up and down about ten pounds throughout her adult years, and she never seemed able to get rid of that last five pounds, even when she was at her slimmest.

Carolyn's father and two of her grandparents had died of heart disease, so she had long tried to eat less fat and exercise when she could. As she moved further into her post-menopausal years Carolyn became even more worried about suffering a heart attack, so she went in for regular checkups and religiously followed her doctor's advice.

After her last exam, Carolyn's doctor told her that her cholesterol had inched up into the danger zone, and that her blood glucose level had moved into the "somewhat high range." He wasn't particularly worried about the five excess pounds currently plaguing Carolyn. He was more concerned about her cholesterol level, and encouraged her to eat less fat and more carbohydrate. To help her do so, he had his nurse give the worried woman a diet that replaced saturated fat with carbohydrate. She was to try it for three months and then return for more complete blood tests.

During the ensuing three months, Carolyn followed her doctor's diet faithfully. When she paid her next visit to the doctor, she was pleased to find that her cholesterol had fallen somewhat, but dismayed that her triglycerides were way too high at 210, while her HDL cholesterol was dangerously low at 35. Neither Carolyn nor her doctor realized that she had Syndrome X, and that her new diet had actually made her condition worse.

If you have Syndrome X, replacing the fat in your diet with carbohydrate will always exacerbate the problem, unless you are losing weight at the same time. (Weight loss helps counterbalance the high glucose/high insulin problem by making your tissues more sensitive to insulin.) Carolyn had Syndrome X but wasn't losing weight, so the diet her doctor recommended increased her insulin and triglyceride levels, while depressing her "good" HDL cholesterol.

A few days after getting the bad news from her physician, a friend suggested to Carolyn that she go to a clinic at Stanford University because "they have a new way of looking at heart disease." The concerned woman did so, becoming even more worried when her new doctor told her that she had Syndrome X. "But," he assured her, "we can do something about it." The diet he gave her was easy to follow and, to Carolyn's relief, quite tasty because it had more fat than she was used to eating. A month later she went back to the Stanford doctor and was delighted to hear that her blood tests were significantly improved.

"My HDL cholesterol increased and my triglycerides fell," she explained. "And it's easy to stay on my diet when I eat out or at a friend's house. I have a lot more freedom to eat what I like while decreasing my chances of having a heart attack at the same time. It's like having my life back."

Imagine a diet that's thoroughly enjoyable and easy to follow, lowers both elevated insulin and high LDL cholesterol levels, and can be used for either weight loss or maintenance. There is such a diet—the Syndrome X Diet™.

The key to this diet is the ratio of protein, fat and carbohydrate (15:40:45) and the kind of fat that's consumed (mostly unsaturated). Here's how the diet breaks down:

Protein	15%
Fat:	40%
Polyunsaturated and monounsaturated fats	30–35%
Saturated fats	5–10%
Carbohydrate	45%

The two-step rationale behind this clinically tested approach is amazingly simple. First, insulin levels do not increase when you eat fat. Whether saturated or unsaturated, fat has no effect on insulin levels. Eat more, eat less, your insulin levels won't budge. However, if you substitute fat for carbohydrate, your insulin levels will fall. This means that, to a certain degree, more fat is good for those with Syndrome X. But not any fat will do, and that brings us to the second point: Unsaturated fats don't raise LDL cholesterol levels. Substituting saturated fat for carbohydrate, bite for bite, will keep your insulin under control but will elevate your "bad" LDL cholesterol. That's dangerous, whether you have Syndrome X or not. And that's why this diet carefully replaces carbohydrate with unsaturated fats. These "good" fats keep insulin *and* LDL under control, which means that this approach guards against the "new" kind of heart disease caused by Syndrome X as well as the "old" kind associated with elevated LDL. You win both ways.

Substituting unsaturated fat for carbohydrate is an easy change for most people to make, since it requires no special foods or cooking techniques. And it's a tasty change for those accustomed to low-fat diets. Fat, after all, tastes good. Most Americans are already eating something very close to the Syndrome X Diet's proportion of protein, fat and carbohydrate. It's simply a matter of adjusting the fat intake, plus replacing some carbohydrate and most of the saturated fat with "good" fats.

The beauty of this scientifically proven diet is that there's nothing "magical," exotic or complicated about it. It seems quite ordinary, for the changes you are asked to make are subtle; a little more of this, a little less of that, eating one type of fat instead of another. Don't be dismayed by the diet's simplicity, for it works, and works well. Instead, enjoy the fact that it's so easy, ordinary and tasty, you'll have no trouble sticking to it for life.

Even if You Don't Need to Lose Weight, You Will Benefit

As part of the full Six-Step Syndrome X Program, this is the only diet that will help reduce or eliminate all of Syndrome X's manifestations.

Whether you have a "mild" or "full-blown" case, this diet is for you.

Whether you're slim, pudgy or obese, this program is for you.

Even if you can't or don't want to shed an ounce, the Syndrome X diet will still help reduce your risk of heart disease.

If you are overweight but are willing and able to slim down, that's even better.

Whether your weight is normal, you're overweight and losing, or are overweight and holding steady, the 15:40:45 Syndrome X Diet will help you:

- Reduce elevated insulin levels
- Lower elevated triglycerides
- Raise HDL "good" cholesterol
- Speed the clearance of fat from your blood following meals
- Eliminate the problem of smaller, denser LDL particles
- Lower LDL "bad" cholesterol

It also stands to reason that the diet will help reduce the formation of unnecessary blood clots, improve your body's ability to dispose of blood clots and may even help return elevated blood pressure to normal. These theoretical benefits, however, have not yet been scientifically demonstrated.

This diet combats all of the Syndrome X risk factors at once. And it's the only diet that can.

Beware Fad Diets

There are too many popular diets to count: diets devised by doctors and laypeople, diets based on blood type or body build, diets that guarantee you'll lose "X" pounds and look great in a bikini. It's best to skip these programs if you have Syndrome X, simply because they are not designed to deal with insulin resistance and compensatory hyperinsulinemia. In fact, many are downright dangerous for people with the syndrome—including some diets that otherwise improve heart health. Take, for example, the American Heart Association diet, The Zone and the Atkins diet.

The highly regarded American Heart Association Diet aims to reduce the risk of heart disease by cutting back on foods high in saturated fat and cholesterol. The program does lower cholesterol levels and is nutritionally balanced, although not so easy to follow. But the good news ends there, for this is the worst kind of diet for people with Syndrome X. A whopping 55 to 60 percent of its calories comes from insulin-stimulating carbohydrate. Another 15 percent comes from protein, which also triggers insulin secretion. You get a total of 70 to 75 percent of your calories from carbohydrate and protein, a tremendous load for your insulin-resistant cells to grapple with. This guarantees that your pancreas will be pumping out more and more insulin, and that your risk of heart attack will rise. If your only concern is lowering cholesterol, this program is probably good for you. But if you have Syndrome X, it can be deadly.

On Barry Sears's The Zone diet, you get 40 percent of your calories from carbohydrate and 30 percent from protein, making it just as dangerous for those with Syndrome X as the American Heart Association diet. The real difference between The Zone diet and the American Heart Association diet is that the former is harder to follow; it takes a lot of planning and requires numerous adjustments for most people. It's also difficult to eat all the suggested protein without taking in a lot of saturated fat in the process. Saturated fat, of course, raises LDL cholesterol and increases the risk of heart disease. The Zone tries to overcome the potential problems of the American Heart Association diet by shifting carbohydrate calories to protein calories. Unfortunately, protein also increases insulin secretion. Why trade one insulin-raising nutrient for another? It is far safer—and just as nutritious—to decrease carbohydrate and maintain protein at a reasonable level, while increasing your intake of the "good" unsaturated fats.

The Atkins diet, which has been around for many, many years, is based on the idea that carbohydrates are bad but everything else is terrific. Bring on the steak, eggs, cheese and butter, says Dr. Atkins. Hold the bread or anything else with carbohydrate! With only 40 percent of its calories coming from carbohydrate and protein combined, the Dr. Atkins Diet can actually be an effective treatment for Syndrome X. After all, 60 percent of its calories comes from fat, which does not stimulate insulin production. Unfortunately, the diet is bad for the heart for other reasons. If the 60 percent fat calories were low in saturated fat, and if the diet were still nutritionally balanced, it would work well for Syndrome Xers. No such luck. The Atkins Diet sample menus and recipes contain roughly 25 percent artery-clogging saturated fat and are loaded with cholesterol.

The Syndrome X Diet, as part of the full six-step program, is the only eating plan that attacks the root causes of the syndrome. With 15

Can a High-Protein Diet Decrease Risk of Heart Attack?

If you have Syndrome X, a high-protein diet can help decrease your risk of heart attack if and only if you lose excess weight and keep it off, and if the diet is low in saturated fat. High-protein diets become troublesome when you aren't losing weight, regardless of how fat or thin you may be to begin with.

Actively losing weight on *any* diet improves your insulin sensitivity. (With greater sensitivity you need less insulin to help transfer glucose into your cells and out of your bloodstream.) As long as you're in the process of losing weight, a high-protein, low-fat diet probably does you no harm. But if you don't lose weight on a high-protein, low-fat diet, or if you lose the desired amount of weight and then hold steady, a high-protein diet can elevate the insulin levels in your blood just as surely as a low-fat, high-carbohydrate diet. And once insulin levels increase, all the manifestations of Syndrome X get worse.

---

percent protein, 40 percent fat (mostly unsaturated) and 45 percent carbohydrate, the eating regimen simultaneously lowers all major risk factors for heart attack. Not only that, it's easy to stick with. Most diets are difficult to stay on for long because they don't let us eat what we like, or they severely restrict calories and leave us feeling deprived. The scientifically tested Syndrome X Diet is easy to follow and requires little planning. With its generous allotment of "good" fats, it satisfies virtually everyone's taste.

The Syndrome X Diet™ Versus the AHA, Zone and Atkins Diets

	Protein	Saturated Fat	Mono & Polyunsaturated Fat	Carbohydrate	Cholesterol	Decreases Both Insulin and LDL Cholesterol
Syndrome X Diet	15%	5–10%	30–35%	45%	<300 mg/day	YES
American Heart Association Diet	15%	5–10%	20%	55–60%	300 mg/day	No
The Zone Diet*	30%	6%	24%	40%	210 mg/day	No
Atkins Diet*	22%	25%	35%	18%	880 mg/day	No

* This diet makes no specific recommendations; recommended menu plans were used to calculate proportions.

DELVING INTO THE DIET

The 15:40:45 ratio of protein to fat to carbohydrate is the key to the Syndrome X Diet. Most of the fat is unsaturated; just a little is saturated. You'll find menus for two full thirty-day diets, one offering 1,800 calories a day and the other 1,200, as well as suggestions for snacks, in the final chapters. For now, let's take a look at fat, cholesterol and tips for eating out. If you're not overweight, combine what you learn in this chapter with the menus, and you'll be all set. If you need to lose weight, study Chapter 7 as well.

A Few Words About Fat

Saturated fat, unsaturated fat, polyunsaturated fat, fatty acids, triglycerides: fat is a pretty meaty subject. Fortunately, the concepts are all simple.

Fat begins with carbon, a very common element found in our bodies, in our food and elsewhere. Each carbon atom has four "hands," and each hand wants to grab onto something.

Imagine a line or a chain of carbon atoms ten, fifteen or more carbons long. The carbons are all neatly lined up, one after the other. With one "hand" each carbon holds on to the one in front of it, and with a second hand each grabs ahold of the carbon behind. That leaves each carbon atom with two "hands" free, but not for long. With each of their two free "hands," the carbons grab hold of hydrogen atoms, holding them off to the side. Everything is in balance: many carbon atoms in a line, each holding on to the carbon in front, the carbon in back, one hydrogen atom to one side, another hydrogen to the other. Add a few miscellaneous atoms to the front and rear of the carbon chain to give the first and last carbons something to fill their hands, and you've got a fatty acid.

Just as amino acids are the building blocks of protein, fatty acids are the stuff fat is made from. There are many different fatty acids, differentiated according to whether or not all the carbons are holding on to two hydrogens, which ones are not, and how many carbons are in the "line."

If each carbon, except the two on the ends, is grasping two hydrogens, it's a saturated fatty acid. All of its "hands" are full; it can't hold any more. But sometimes two carbons standing next to each other will each "let go" of a hydrogen. When that happens, the fatty acid is no longer saturated; it could hold more hydrogens. If one pair does this, the fatty acid is monounsaturated (mono = one). If more than one pair does this, the fatty acid is polyunsaturated (poly = many). So the difference between saturated, monounsaturated and polyunsaturated fats comes down to who's holding whose hand.

As groups, the saturated, polyunsaturated and monounsaturated fats have different effects on the body:

- Saturated fats, found primarily in meat, butter, cheese, lard and other foods that come from animals, raise total cholesterol and "bad" LDL cholesterol levels.
- Polyunsaturated fats, found in corn, soybean and safflower oil, help lower LDL cholesterol.
- Monounsaturated fats, found in olive, canola and peanut oil, also help lower LDL cholesterol. At the same time, they may protect LDL cholesterol from being oxidized, a dangerous process that encourages the buildup of plaque on artery walls and can lead to heart attacks.

Saturated, polyunsaturated and monounsaturated fats of different lengths are building blocks that can be combined, separated and recombined in the body as necessary. Quite often, the body attaches three fatty acids to a glycerol molecule, forming a triglyceride (tri = three). This is what we typically think of when referring to blood fats.

There's nothing wrong with fat per se; it provides essential nutrition, helps cushion certain body structures and serves as a concentrated form of stored energy. It's only when we have too much of it on our bodies, or eat too much of the wrong kind, that we get into trouble.

We need to eat a fair amount of the "good" unsaturated fat every day, and can certainly tolerate a small amount of "bad" saturated fat. Most government agencies and health organizations are overly simplistic when they recommend that we eat less fat. This advice does not take into account the type of fat that should be restricted, or what will replace that fat in the diet. This recommendation needs to be updated to address the needs of those at risk of heart attacks due to Syndrome X, type 2 diabetes or hypertension. The solution that will work for everyone is decreasing the saturated fat in our diets and replacing it with "good" (unsaturated) fat, instead of carbohydrate. That's just what the Syndrome X Diet does.

Finding the Fat

All diets contain saturated, polyunsaturated and monounsaturated fats. It's very difficult to avoid any one type, because they tend to be found in combination. When we say that a certain food is a source of saturated fat, we don't mean that it contains *only* saturated fat—most likely it contains some unsaturated fat as well. For example, more than 60 percent of the fatty acids in butter fat are saturated, so it's referred to as a source of saturated fat. But it also has polyunsaturated and monounsaturated fats. Corn oil, on the other hand, is about 60 percent polyunsaturated fat, 25 percent monounsaturated fat and 15 percent saturated. Despite the presence of some saturated fat, we generally refer to corn oil as a source of unsaturated fat.

As a general rule, you'll find saturated fats in meat, milk, butter, cheese, palm oil and coconut oil. Here's another tip: the harder a fat is at room temperature, the more saturated it is. Cheese and the fat on steak, both of which will remain solid at room temperature, are quite heavily saturated, while the fat in vegetable oils, which are liquid at room temperature, are mostly unsaturated. Different "versions" of the same food can also contain widely variable amounts of saturated fat. The hard stick margarines, for example, contain much more saturated fat than do soft "diet" margarines.

It's not always obvious which foods are saturated and which are not, so here are three lists to help you choose foods wisely:

Foods High in Saturated ("Hard") Fat
The fat on or in meat, poultry, eggs
Bacon
Banana chips
Bologna, salami luncheon meats
Butter
Cheese
Chocolate
Cream
Cream cheese
Coconut or coconut oil
Fatback or salt pork
Fried foods
Ice cream
Lard

Milk, whole
Palm and palm kernel oil
Shortening and stick margarines

Foods Low in Saturated Fat
Avocado
Fish
Margarine, soft or liquid
Mayonnaise
Milk products, nonfat
Nuts, most varieties
Oils (canola, corn, olive, safflower, peanut, soybean, sunflower)
Olives
Peanuts and peanut butter
Seeds (pumpkin, sesame, sunflower)
Turkey and chicken, white meat without skin, broiled or grilled

Foods with Little or No Saturated Fat
Beans, dried
Candy, hard
Fruits
Grains
Juices
Pasta
Soft drinks
Sugars
Vegetables

Margarine: Is It Better Than Butter?

We know butter is bad for heart health because it's loaded with saturated fat. But what about margarine? Margarine has been around since World War II, when its pale appearance brought to mind small bricks of lard, and one had to mix in yellow food coloring to make it look more appetizing. Not only did early margarine look like lard, it was just about as unhealthy, loaded with saturated fat, while packing the same amount of calories as butter.

Luckily, manufacturers today produce much improved margarines. Made from monounsaturated and polyunsaturated oils, they are virtually cholesterol free, and the softer tub margarines contain as little as 1.2 grams of saturated fat per tablespoon. Better yet, the liquid margarines that come in squeeze bottles have half as much saturated fat as tub margarines. Compared to butter, which contains 7.6 grams of saturated fat and 33 milligrams of cholesterol per tablespoon, margarine is a boon to those concerned about heart disease.

The margarine you select, however, is very important, for not all margarines are equally beneficial. In order to make vegetable oil into something with the approximate firmness and spreadability of butter, manufacturers must transform the healthy mono- and polyunsaturated oils through a process called hydrogenation. Manufacturers do so because the margarine will then remain solid at room temperature and will melt at a higher temperature than before. And if you combine it with flour to make a piecrust, you'll get a flaky product rather than a messy, oily one.

Unfortunately, hydrogenation has two major unhealthy side effects. As hydrogen gas is added to the liquid oil, the process changes the chemical structure of the oil so that it behaves more like artery-clogging saturated fat. The second health risk the hydrogenation process creates is the transformation of fatty acids, from what is known as a "cis" shape to a "trans" shape. These trans-fatty acids increase the amount of heart-damaging LDL cholesterol, while simultaneously decreasing the amount of heart-protective HDL cholesterol.

Not all margarines are hydrogenated to the same extent. You can tell which are the most hydrogenated just by looking: the firmer the product, the more it's been hydrogenated. Margarine that comes in a cube contains more hydrogenated fat than margarine that comes in a tub. The least hydrogenated margarine is the liquid kind that comes in a squeeze bottle. You can also check the list of ingredients on the packaging. Although all margarines contain a certain amount of hydrogenated oil, look for ones with monounsaturated and polyunsaturated oils as a primary ingredient—or, even better, as the first ingredient. The best test of a healthful margarine is to determine the ratio of mono- and polyunsaturated (good) fats to saturated (bad) fat. The higher the ratio of good fats to saturated fat, the better the margarine will be for you. (Be sure to watch your intake of fast food, since fast-food chains commonly precook their food in hydrogenated shortening loaded with trans-fatty acids. An occasional fast-food meal won't harm you, but a steady diet of fast food certainly can.)

So which is better: butter, with its saturated fat and cholesterol, or margarine, with its hydrogenated fat and trans-fatty acids? There is no simple answer, but there are some easy-to-follow guidelines. The harder the margarine and the greater the amount of saturated fat it contains, the less healthy it will be compared to butter. At the other extreme are soft and liquid margarines, all of which are less hydrogenated and contain primarily monounsaturated and polyunsaturated fats. These margarines are much healthier choices than butter, and there are now some brands that are trans fat free. There is also a new margarine on the market called Benecol which has actually been shown to lower LDL cholesterol somewhat. However, Benecol is still very expensive and is not, by itself, a particularly effective way to lower cholesterol. If price is not important, there is no reason you shouldn't use Benecol. On the other hand, the benefit of using Benecol, compared to much less expensive soft margarines, free of trans fats, may not be very great.

Even healthier for you than any margarine on the market today are olive oil and other monounsaturated and polyunsaturated fats. Breads and crackers dipped into these oils—after you add a few seasonings such as rosemary or a dash of dried pepper flakes—can be very tasty. Many people like these seasoned oils even better than margarine.

Eating Less Cholesterol

Most people are concerned about their total cholesterol levels, and try to control them by eating fewer cholesterol-containing foods. That's not a bad idea, but restricting these foods will not lower elevated insulin levels. Furthermore, the quantity of cholesterol-rich food you consume has much less effect on your LDL cholesterol levels than does saturated fat.

How much cholesterol you can safely eat will depend on your current cholesterol levels, other heart attack risk factors and how cholesterol-sensitive you are. Since most of us have no idea how cholesterol-sensitive we are, and since the foods that contain cholesterol also tend to contain saturated fat, cutting back on your cholesterol intake is probably a prudent idea. To be safe, limit your intake to no more than 150 milligrams per 1,000 calories eaten per day. If you're taking in 2,000 calories a day, you can safety eat 300 milligrams of cholesterol, approximately the amount found in an egg. Here is a brief list of foods high in cholesterol to watch out for:

Food	Serving	Mg, Cholesterol
Beef kidney	1 ounce	110
Beef liver	1 ounce	86
Bernaise or hollandaise sauce	1 cup	189
Bologna lunch meats	1 slice	52
Cheddar cheese	1 ounce	30
Chicken liver	1 ounce	180
Clams, canned	1 cup	101
Crab, fresh cooked	1 cup, unpacked	125
Cream, whipping, light	1 cup	265
Egg yolk, medium	1 whole	270
Hamburger, Big Mac	4 ounces	107
Ice cream, regular	1 cup	59
Lobster, cooked	1 cup	123
Milk, whole	1 cup	33
Noodles, egg	1 cup	50
Oysters, raw	1 cup	120
Quiche Lorraine	1/8 of pie	235
Sausage, Polish	1 link	47
Shrimp, canned	1 cup	192
Sweetbreads, beef	1 ounce	132
Turkey bologna or hot dogs	1 ounce	37

These foods are either low in cholesterol or cholesterol-free:

Avocado
Beans
Breads, plain
Carbonated beverages
Cereals, dry and cooked
Canola oil
Coffee
Corn oil
Egg white
Egg substitute
Fig bars
Fruits
Gelatin
Ginger snaps

Grains
Honey
Juices
Liquor and wine
Milk (skim, nonfat, low-fat, low-fat buttermilk)
Molasses
Olive oil
Peanut oil
Safflower oil
Soybean oil
Sunflower oil
Pasta
Peanut butter
Rice
Sugar, white and brown
Syrup, cane and maple
Tapioca, dry
Tea
Vegetables

As you may have noticed, cholesterol is only found in foods that come from animals (meat, milk, fish, etc.). If a food grows in or out of the ground, or on a bush, vine or tree, it contains absolutely no cholesterol. As a rule of thumb, when you avoid cholesterol, you will also cut back on your intake of saturated fats.

Eating Out

Eating out occasionally is not a major issue. What you consume over the long haul will have a major influence on your insulin and LDL cholesterol levels, but a "bad" meal once in a while won't be disastrous, especially if you order wisely most of the time. Eating out often, however, requires a different strategy because it's difficult to know exactly which ingredients restaurants use in their dishes, and how many calories or grams of fat you're getting in a meal. A recent study completed for the National Health and Nutrition Examination Survey found that even trained dietitians had difficulty estimating the amount of fat and calories in restaurant foods accurately, from hamburgers to Caesar salad.

Despite the difficulties, you can limit the harm that may come from eating out. Here are some tips:

- *Choosing the restaurant*—You'll find your best food choices in seafood restaurants, grills, steak houses with grilled chicken and fish, salad bars, stir-fry places that use the "good" polyunsaturated or monounsaturated fats or any establishment with such cuisine.
- *Breakfast*—Avoid anything fried or made with whole milk or cheese. Watch out for scrambled eggs made with unidentified kinds of fat. Instead of a sticky bun, order a poached or soft-boiled egg, English muffin, bagel or toast. Ask for soft margarine instead of cream cheese and butter. Dry or cooked cereals with fresh fruit and low-fat milk are usually healthy choices, if you avoid the sugary "kid" cereals.
- *Main courses*—Broiled or grilled fish and chicken top the list of good choices, but hold the sauces. Pasta with garlic and olive oil is an excellent selection; so are any fresh vegetable stir-fried dishes made with polyunsaturated and monounsaturated oils, with or without meat or fish. Don't be afraid to ask which dishes are lowest in fat, or what kind of fat the chef uses. If you order a dish high in saturated fat, or if it comes in an extra-large portion, either share the dish with a friend or save half of it for lunch the next day.
- *Vegetables and side dishes*—Go for stir-fried or steamed fresh vegetables, a baked potato, steamed rice or other grains. Reach for the olive oil instead of creamy sauces or sour cream. If a dish comes with sauce, order the sauce on the side so you can control how much you eat. Try vinaigrette salad dressing on potatoes, vegetables or other foods.
- *Salads*—Green salad with vinaigrette dressing is a good choice. Pile on the tomatoes, garbanzo beans, green beans and chilled asparagus if you want, but skip the cheese.
- *Bread*—Any plain bread is fine. To moisten it, dip it in olive oil or spread with safflower margarine.
- *Dessert*—A rich dessert now and then isn't going to do you in. However, the best choice is plain fresh fruit.

What about fast food? (Is "healthy fast food" an oxymoron?) Eating one or two meals in a fast-food restaurant probably won't be too harmful to your health, especially since there are usually a few good choices on the menu. But a word to the wise: many fast-food restaurants get precooked or partially cooked food from factories that use lard or other saturated fats because they're cheaper. When the food arrives at the restaurant, it may be drenched in saturated fat yet again. (Batter-prepared or fried chicken is often one of these "factory foods.") Even if the restaurant advertises that it uses "good" fat, the factory probably doesn't.

Still, by paying attention to the guidelines below, you can eat at fast-food restaurants once in a while and still follow the Syndrome X Diet.

Poor Fast-Food Choices	Better Fast-Food Choices
Creamy dressings	Oil and vinegar dressing
Deep-fried foods	Roast beef sandwich on whole wheat bread
Hamburger or hot dog	Grilled chicken on a bun or baked potato
Fried fish sandwich	Sliced turkey breast sandwich
Whole milk	Low-fat milk or diet soft drink
Milkshake	Low-fat chocolate milk, diet soft drinks
Onion rings	Coleslaw
Taco shells or tortilla chips	Pretzels or English muffin
Salad with cheesy croutons	Salad with chicken or shrimp
Brownies, cookies, pies	Low-fat yogurt

DIETARY FALLACIES

Using what you've learned here, plus the menus in Chapters 15 and 16, you'll soon be all set to embark on the Syndrome X Diet. There may be some bumps and detours along the way; you may find your resolution wavering, or you may occasionally eat the wrong foods. Don't worry if that happens. Resolve to do better and stick to the program. And beware of these dietary fallacies:

Fallacy #1: Obesity causes insulin resistance.

Obesity does not cause insulin resistance. Not all obese people are insulin resistant, and not everyone with Syndrome X is obese. Your genetic inheritance from your parents is the single most powerful factor to consider, while differences in weight account for no more than one-quarter of the differences in insulin action from person to person. However, obesity does make insulin resistance worse. Just losing ten or fifteen pounds can dramatically increase your insulin sensitivity and reduce your coronary heart disease risk factors. In fact, in certain cases just losing excess weight is enough to overcome *all* of the symptoms of Syndrome X.

We haven't yet tracked down each and every link between obesity and Syndrome X, but it seems that elevated fatty acid levels in the blood interfere with the ability of insulin to stimulate the movement of glucose into the muscle cells. Plasma fatty acids are higher in obese individuals, probably because they have greater amounts of fatty tissue. Losing excess weight decreases the level of fatty acids and increases the ability of insulin to stimulate glucose uptake.

Fallacy #2: Calories don't count.

Many people believe that they can eat as much as they want without getting fat *if* they eat the right kinds or the right combinations of foods. For example, the popular 1970s grapefruit-bacon-and-eggs diet allowed you to eat all you wanted of these three foods, as long as you consumed all three in the same sitting, and ate them at every meal. Despite the claims, any weight lost on this "diet" had nothing to do with a "magic" combination of foods. You lost weight simply because you got so tired of grapefruit, bacon and eggs that you ate less in the long run!

There are no special combinations of foods that guarantee weight loss, no way to combine foods so that the calories in one "erase" those in another. A calorie is a calorie is a calorie, whether it comes from a banana, a chocolate bar, a carrot or glass of beer. A hot fudge sundae may have more calories per mouthful than a carrot, but the individual calories from each provide equal amounts of energy.

Unglamorous as it sounds, all weight loss is the result of a very simple equation: more calories must be expended than ingested. If you take in fewer calories than you burn, you'll lose weight. If you take in more calories than you burn, you'll gain weight. Calories count. To lose weight, eat less and exercise more. It's as simple as that.

> ### Different Numbers, Same Result
>
> It's true that a gram of fat contains 9 calories, while carbohydrates and protein only have 4 calories per gram. If you look only at grams, fat appears to be more fattening than carbohydrate or protein. But the calories in carbohydrate or protein provide just as much energy, and exactly as much potential for weight gain, as the calories in fat. There are more calories in fat, ounce for ounce, but there's nothing magical about them.

Fallacy #3: My metabolism won't let me lose weight.

Variations in metabolic rate have relatively little do to with weight gain or loss. There are small differences in the amount of energy people get when they metabolize food; some may be able to get "more energy per bite" than others. However, current scientific studies all indicate that the differences are slight and not enough to account for much weight gain. Of course, even small differences in energy utilization can lead to significant weight gain over the long haul. Suppose, for example, Steven and Mark both ingest 2,000 calories per day, and their energy outputs are identical. If Steven is 4 percent more efficient at "getting" calories from his food, he's receiving the equivalent of 80 additional calories per day. It's as if his diet contains 2,080 calories per day, compared to Mark's 2,000. Eighty calories per day times 365 days equals 29,200 "extra" calories a year for Steven. That sounds like a big problem for the poor guy until you consider that he could erase the "additional calories" by eating one less piece of bread a day.

Fallacy #4: My genes make me fat.

Over the last few years, newspapers have carried sensational stories describing newly discovered genes that are supposedly responsible for obesity, Alzheimer's disease, alcoholism, schizophrenia, sexual orientation, and other ailments, conditions and orientations. Usually, way down toward the end of the article, you read that the genes in question only play a small role. Moreover, the conclusions are often based on studies with mice, so their findings may or may not be relevant to humans.

Not too many years ago, researchers announced the discovery of several genes for obesity in mice. One of these is tied to a protein called leptin, which is believed to inhibit appetite. Most strains of mice secrete leptin from their fat tissues: releasing more would curb the little animal's appetites, releasing less would make them hungrier. At least one study has shown that a particular strain of genetically obese mice lacks the ability to make leptin and so they eat almost constantly.

But the story doesn't end there. Humans also make leptin in their fat tissues. It's released into the bloodstream, where it is quite easy to measure. Based on the mouse studies, it may be tempting to conclude that human obesity is also caused by a lack of leptin. But researchers found that just the opposite is true: the overwhelming majority of obese people have *higher* levels of leptin in their blood. And the heavier they are, the more blood leptin. However, a few patients who are not producing leptin at all have also been identified. They are massively obese and, like the mice, have insatiable appetites. Their degree of obesity and their compulsive eating behavior easily distinguish them from the rest of us.

There is some evidence that there are leptin receptors in the human appetite center. If these receptors don't recognize leptin when they are supposed to, even high blood levels of this protein won't signal people to stop eating. If that's true, those with defective leptin receptors may eat more and gain more weight, and their increased mass of fat tissue may put out more and more leptin, explaining the increased levels in the blood. If that's so, "leptin resistance" in the appetite center would cause obesity. Then again, it's just as likely that leptin has nothing to do with weight gain in most people. The elevated leptin levels in the bloodstreams of the obese may simply reflect the fact that they have more fat tissue to release the protein.

Genetic effects over weight gain/loss are not very powerful, and most likely do not account for more than a 4 percent difference in energy efficiency. Compensating for this minor difference is not that difficult; consuming one less slice of bread or can of cola per day just about covers it.

Fallacy #5: Low-fat diets make you skinny, and high-carbohydrate diets make you fat.

Eating less fat has long been prescribed as the way to lose weight. This approach works, but not because fat is sinister. Fat is the most concentrated source of calories, so cutting back on fat automatically ensures a cutback in calories. But that only works if you don't replace the fat calories with calories from protein and carbohydrate. If you eat less fat but take in even more calories in the form of carbohydrate or protein, you will gain weight.

By the same token, increasing your carbohydrate intake may lead to higher insulin levels, but that doesn't automatically mean you'll gain weight. Insulin does not make you gain weight—taking in excess calories does. Contrary to what many people believe, bread and potatoes aren't "fattening" in and of themselves. They're like other foods; if you eat too much of them, your caloric intake will exceed your body's needs and you'll gain weight. Remember, weight is a reflection of energy intake versus energy output, or calories in versus calories out. Good health, however, depends on fulfilling those energy needs by consuming a wide variety of healthful foods.

Fallacy #6: High-protein diets make it easy to lose weight.

Several popular diet books claim that high-protein diets help you lose weight because they lower insulin levels. They also claim that switching from carbohydrates to protein will help you avoid the perils of elevated insulin. Unfortunately, *Protein Power*, *The Zone* and other pop diet and weight loss books have hijacked and badly mangled the research we've conducted at Stanford University. Their interpretation of our research findings is more fiction than fact.

Let's begin with the assertion that eating more protein and less carbohydrate will cause you to secrete less insulin. It's not true. We know that protein is broken down into amino acids during digestion, and that amino acids stimulate the pancreas to release more insulin. As far as insulin production is concerned, swapping carbohydrate for protein is most likely an even trade-off.

As for protein's "magical" ability to make the pounds melt away, remember that a calorie is a calorie, regardless of whether it comes in the form of protein, fat or carbohydrate. If you take in fewer calories than you expend, you will lose weight. Carbohydrates do not, in and of themselves, make you fat. It's a simple matter of calories in versus calories out.

A NOTE ON CALCIUM

It takes a plentiful and steady stream of calcium to build bones when you're young, then maintain them into old age. Ninety-nine percent of the calcium we take in daily goes to developing, maintaining and repairing bone; neither males nor females ever outgrow their need for this mineral. Unfortunately, most Americans don't get enough calcium.

Milk and cheese are very good, very well-known sources of calcium. Some people, however, fearing heart disease, shy away from eating dairy products. It's true that the saturated fat and cholesterol in dairy products can damage arteries. But it's not all bad news. Calcium plays an active role in muscle contraction, nerve transmission and other basic body functions; the body needs sufficient calcium to regulate its heartbeat. Calcium may even play a part in lowering blood pressure.

You'll get about 500 milligrams of calcium a day on the 1,800 calorie Syndrome X Diet. That's not really enough, so take a daily calcium supplement to ensure that you get as much calcium as you need, without sabotaging your heart with saturated fat-laden dairy products.

This table will help you select a calcium tablet supplement based on your age and gender requirements. For example, if you are a female over fifty-one years of age on the Syndrome X Diet, you will need a 1,000 milligram daily elemental calcium supplement in addition to the 500 milligrams of calcium you will get from your food.

Daily Elemental Calcium Requirements

	Male	Female
Age 1 to 10	800 mg	800 mg
Age 11 to 24	1,200 mg	1,200 mg
Age 25 to 50	800 mg	800 mg
Age 51 and over	800 mg	1,500 mg
Pregnant and nursing women		1,200 mg

Heart-Healthy Calcium Sources

Here are some foods high in calcium and low in saturated fat—heart-healthy alternatives to dairy products.

	Calcium	Calories
1 cup nonfat yogurt	450 mg	130
1 cup low-fat yogurt	400 mg	140
1 cup 1% milk	300 mg	102
1 cup 2% milk	297 mg	121
1 cup nonfat milk	302 mg	86
½ cup tofu	130 mg	94
1 cup 1% cottage cheese	138 mg	164
1 cup 2% cottage cheese	155 mg	203
1 cup ice milk	176 mg	184
1 ounce skim mozzarella cheese	183 mg	72
1 cup calcium-fortified orange juice	270 mg	120
½ cup spinach	122 mg	25
½ cup broccoli	55 mg	25
½ cup collard greens	148 mg	27
½ cup kale	47 mg	21
½ cup chard	51 mg	18
1 cup garbanzo beans	80 mg	269
1 cup hummus	124 mg	420
1 cup cooked kidney beans	50 mg	225
1 cup cooked lentils	37 mg	231
1 cup cooked lima beans	32 mg	217

Remember, the Syndrome X Diet is good for you whether you have Syndrome X or not, whether you are trying to lose weight or not. It's especially healthy compared to other popular diets, including The Zone, the American Heart Association diet, the Atkins diet and Protein Power. This is the only diet that will reduce all the manifestations of Syndrome X and lower LDL cholesterol, helping to reduce your risk of heart disease and setting you on the road to great overall health.

SLIMMING

THE SYNDROME

Even if you don't lose an ounce, your insulin and triglyceride levels will fall while you're on the Syndrome X Diet™. That's good. But if you need to lose weight, doing so will make these results even better.

Let's be honest: it isn't always easy to lose weight. It helps to be motivated, to know why you need to lose weight and to have a plan. That's why I'll begin by looking at the scientific evidence proving that weight loss is an excellent "medicine" for Syndrome X. Then I'll show you my four-step formula for permanent weight loss.

LOSING WEIGHT IS MEDICINAL

More than twenty-five years ago, before we had even named the syndrome, our research group published the first paper[1] showing that losing weight is beneficial for controlling both insulin and triglyceride levels. Thirty-six overweight volunteers between the ages of twenty-four and sixty-nine participated in this study. As a group, they were quite insulin resistant. But when they lost an average of twenty pounds in about five months, their insulin efficiency improved by approximately 40 percent.

We measured the glucose and insulin levels in our participants first thing in the morning, before they had eaten, and then gave them

---

[1] J. Olefsky, G. M. Reaven, and J. W. Farquhar. "Effects of weight reduction on obesity." *The Journal of Clinical Investigation*, Vol. 53, January 1974:64–76.

each a drink containing 75 grams of glucose for a glucose tolerance test. Their glucose and insulin levels were measured again at 30, 60, 120, and 180 minutes after they drank this sugary fluid.

The levels of both blood glucose and insulin increased during the first 60 minutes, and returned to the baseline by 180 minutes, both before and after weight loss. Losing weight did not have a dramatic effect on the shape of the glucose response curve, although the absolute values were slightly lower after the participants lost weight.

There was, however, a dramatic change in the insulin curve. The very high insulin concentrations before weight loss, caused by insulin resistance, flattened out considerably as the patients' bellies shrunk. And, in addition, blood triglyceride concentrations fell by more than 100 mg/dl in the thirty-six volunteers.

WEIGHT LOSS, A FOUR-STEP FORMULA

Here's the only "scientific" information you, as a dieter, will need to lay the foundation for successful weight loss: you'll lose weight when you take in fewer calories than you need to maintain your current weight. You'll gain weight when you take in more calories than you need. You'll hold steady when you take in exactly as many calories as you need.

With that in mind, let's look at my four-step formula for permanent weight loss. It's simple. You figure out what it takes to hold your weight steady, decide how many pounds to shed, translate those pounds into the amount of calories you need to skip, then recalculate your caloric needs during the maintenance phase.

Step 1. Figure Out What It Takes to Hold Steady

Begin by figuring out how many calories you need to maintain your current weight. Fortunately, the amount of energy derived from a given amount of food varies very little from person to person, and physical activity really doesn't have that much of an impact on calorie needs. For example, those who are physically inactive may need to consume only 14 calories per pound of body weight to maintain their weight, while very physically active people may need as many as 16 calories per pound to keep their weight stable.[2] The difference is only

[2] The 14, 15 and 16 figures are averages useful for general calculations, and may not apply to children, athletes or pregnant women. Your physician can do more specific calculations for you.

2 calories per pound! (In order to keep it simple, most of the calculations in this chapter will assume you're moderately active and are burning 15 calories per pound of body weight.)

Use these simple calculations to figure out approximately how many calories you must consume daily to hold your weight steady:

If you are fairly inactive at work and play:

_____ × 14 = _____
your current weight   your daily caloric requirement

If you are moderately active:

_____ × 15 = _____
your current weight   your daily caloric requirement

If you are fairly active at work and/or play:

_____ × 16 = _____
your current weight   your daily caloric requirement

You can also use this table, which is based on 15 calories per pound of body weight, to approximate your daily caloric requirements:

Current Weight	Calories Needed to Maintain Your Weight
100	1,500
110	1,650
120	1,800
130	1,950
140	2,100
150	2,250
160	2,400
170	2,550
180	2,700
190	2,880
200	3,000
210	3,150
220	3,300
230	3,450
240	3,600
250	3,750

The simple formulas and the table above are accurate enough for most people. If you are very active or inactive, if you are still growing, if you are pregnant, lactating or ill, or if you want to calculate your daily calorie needs down to the last decimal, see your physician or a registered dietitian.

Step 2. Decide How Many Pounds to Shed

Discuss your weight with your doctor and figure out how many pounds you need to lose. (You can calculate your ideal body mass index by following the simple formula in Chapter 11, but don't fixate on theoretical models of perfection. It's great to have a long-term goal, but remember that just losing weight, no matter how little, can help you immensely.)

As a general rule, it's best to lose no more than one to two pounds per week. Yes, you can lose more by following a "crash diet," but your health may crash as well if you're not careful to get all the nutrients you need. And losing more than two pounds a week probably means you're losing water and/or muscle, two things you need to keep. A one-to-two-pound weight loss each week is enough to make you feel like you're making great progress, which you are, but not so much that the diet becomes difficult or dangerous.

Step 3. Translate Pounds into the Amount of Calories You Need to Skip

Now that you know how many calories you need to maintain your weight, the next step is figuring out how many you need to skip in order to lose weight.

By limiting weight loss to one or two pounds a week, you can be confident that the weight you lose will come from your fat stores, rather than from muscle or water. There are approximately 3,500 calories' worth of energy in one pound of stored body fat. So, to lose one pound you must take in a total of 3,500 fewer calories than your body needs.

Suppose that you weigh 170 pounds and your activity level is average and unchanging. Your daily calorie requirement is 2,550 calories (170 pounds times 15 calories per pound). Now you go on a weight-loss diet providing 1,800 calories per day. Every day on the program, you're in negative caloric balance to the tune of 750 calories (2,550 calories to maintain your weight, minus 1,800 calories for weight loss, or 750 calories). It should take you approximately 4.5

days to lose one pound (3,500 calories divided by 750 calories fewer per day comes to 4.7 days). On this regimen you could lose 20 pounds in about 90 days.

Now suppose that you weigh 170 pounds, that your activity level is average and steady, and you go on a 2,000-calorie-per-day diet. You need 2,550 calories per day to maintain your weight, so you're "losing" 550 calories daily. At that rate it will take you 6.4 days to lose one pound (3,500 divided by 550), and 130 days to lose 20 pounds.

The nearby table, based on 15 calories per pound of body weight, shows how many calories you should consume daily in order to drop about two pounds per week.

Calories for Ideal Weight Loss

Your Current Weight	Calories Needed to Maintain That Weight	Calories Consumed On Weight-Loss Diet	Weekly Weight Loss (Approximate)
140 lbs	2,100	1,200	1.8 lbs.
150 lbs	2,250	1,200	2.1 lbs.
160 lbs	2,400	1,500	1.8 lbs.
170 lbs	2,550	1,500	2.1 lbs.
180 lbs	2,700	1,800	1.8 lbs.
190 lbs	2,850	1,800	2.1 lbs.
200 lbs	3,000	2,100	1.8 lbs.
210 lbs	3,150	2,100	2.1 lbs.

Remember: it doesn't matter how long it takes you to lose the weight. The goal is to lose weight safely and to keep it off forever.

Step 4. Recalculate Your Caloric Needs for Maintenance Purposes

"I've lost the weight, but now what? What do I eat to make sure I don't regain it?" That's a good question and, fortunately, a simple one to answer. Once you've dropped down to your target weight, you'll need to eat just enough calories to hold steady.

Remember that it takes an average of 15 calories per pound to maintain weight. If you weighed 170 before you began your diet, you were probably eating 2,550 calories per day (170 pounds times 15 calories per pound).

After five months' diligent dieting, you weigh 150 pounds. To hold steady, you'll need to consume 2,250 calories per day (150 × 15 calories per pound).

In other words, you can eat 88 percent as much as you did when you weighed 170 pounds and still maintain your current weight.

Plug your new weight into the calculation aids to figure out approximately how many calories you must consume daily to hold your weight steady:

If you are fairly inactive at work and play:

_____ × 14 = _____
your new weight   your daily caloric "steady state" requirement

If you are moderately active:

_____ × 15 = _____
your new weight   your daily caloric "steady state" requirement

If you are fairly active at work and/or play:

_____ × 16 = _____
your new weight   your daily caloric "steady state" requirement

There's the four-step formula for losing weight: figure out what it takes to hold your weight steady, decide how many pounds to shed, translate those pounds into the amount of calories you'll need to skip, and recalculate your caloric needs for maintenance purposes. You're ready to begin losing weight and gaining health.

EXERCISE AND WEIGHT LOSS

So far, all of the calculations have assumed that your level of physical activity remains the same. However, there's no doubt that becoming more active is of great help when you're trying to lose weight. By burning extra calories through exercise, you'll have an easier time controlling your weight, while simultaneously improving your insulin sensitivity.

Suppose you weigh 170 pounds, are moderately active and consume 2,550 calories per day. With that calorie intake and activity level, your weight should hold steady.

Now suppose you keep the same eating and exercise regimen, but add a 30-minute jogging session four days a week. Each session burns up about 300 calories. Four sessions per week burn some 1,200 calories, coming close to 5,000 extra calories burned per month. It only takes a 3,500 calorie deficit to lose a pound of fat tissue. By keeping your calorie intake constant and adding nothing more to your lifestyle than those four sessions per week, you'll burn up 60,000 calories per year, or the equivalent of 17 pounds. And not only will those 17 pounds disappear, your cardiovascular system will become stronger.

MAKING THE LEAP

Despite the claims made by some weight-loss programs, and the talk of blood types, food combining, supplements and "metabolic enhancers," there's nothing terribly complex or mysterious about losing weight. The difficulty most often lies in our inability to commit to an exercise and eating program permanently. It's not easy; we have to establish new habits, we have to learn to think in new ways. It's certainly not impossible, especially if you start one step at a time. And it's probably a lot easier than you think, because on the Syndrome X Diet you'll eat pretty much the way you do now, with only slight modifications.

Here are some tips to help you get started on your health-enhancing diet and stick to it:

- *Emphasize your strongest motivation.* Do you want to lose weight to look better? To be more active? To feel better about yourself? These are all fine goals, but not nearly as powerful as this one: losing weight on the Syndrome X Diet will dramatically reduce your risk of suffering a heart attack, adding years to your life and life to your years. Keep focusing on how much your heart is going to appreciate all you're doing for it. And by the way, you'll also look better, have more energy and feel a lot better about yourself.
- *Figure out what makes you tick.* Many people don't really know what they're eating day in and day out. Before making dramatic changes in your eating habits, try keeping a food diary for a week. Write down everything you eat, estimating portion sizes if you're not sure. And make notes of where you are, what you're feeling and why you're eating. Not only will this little exercise make you aware of what you're eating, it may also reveal some interesting information. You may find that you're taking in more calories than you thought. You may be eating when you're not hungry—out of boredom, anger or frustration. You may be eating more at home than at work, possibly be-

cause you eat while watching television. You may be selecting foods particularly rich in calories because you're always in a rush and it's the most convenient thing to do. Figuring out what makes you tick helps you formulate your strategy.

- *Start easy; you're in it for the long haul.* You may "screw your courage to the sticking post" and dramatically slash your food intake, practically starving as you eat nothing but rice and oranges all day. But after a few days of that, you'll probably throw in the towel and go back to your old ways. That's what happens to most dieters who make major changes in their eating habits; they get discouraged by overly restrictive diets and go back to their old habits, gaining back all the weight they've lost and then some. That's why it's best to start easy and stick with it. The dietary guidelines in this chapter might seem too liberal for veteran dieters, but follow them carefully because an extra doughnut here or a candy bar there could sabotage your chances of losing weight.
- *Eat exclusively.* Make eating your main focus, not a sideline. Sit down at the table when you eat; don't stand over the sink or chow down in the car. Eat what appeals to you, and do nothing but eat. Don't reach for a newspaper, a book or anything else that will make you unaware of what you are eating and why. Forget about the television. Chew slowly and focus on what you're eating. Remember what you're accomplishing by eating so healthfully, and why it makes such a difference. The more you pay attention to these matters, the better your chances of success.
- *Find other ways to attend to your emotional needs.* Who hasn't reached for a cookie instead of tackling a household chore, or gobbled ice cream straight from the carton when upset? "Goodie gobbling" is a quick and easy way to distract, reward or assuage ourselves when we're feeling powerless, tired, bored, lonely, overwhelmed or neglected. Doing so may temporarily quell emotional hunger, but engaging in too much of this behavior makes weight loss nearly impossible.

MENU PLANNING

You now have the tools to maintain your weight and achieve your weight-loss goals, and to put the Syndrome X Diet principles into practice. To help make this final step easier, I've presented two sets of menus in Part Three. Each is for a thirty-day period; one provides 1,200 calories per day, the other 1,800.

Clearly, the best diets are tailored to your specific needs. But since it would be impractical to create thirty-day menus for every conceivable calorie level, I have selected the 1,200 and 1,800 calorie menu plans and given tips for adjusting the calorie content up or down as needed.

Remember that it's best to lose weight at a comfortable pace on a program you can maintain for life. You're in this for years to come. You're a marathon runner, not a sprinter; you've got to set a pace that will carry you for miles and miles, rather than burn out too quickly by trying to race ahead. But don't take the "race" metaphor too literally; this isn't a contest. It doesn't matter when you get to the finish line or how much weight you've lost when you do. If you lose weight (*any* weight) and keep it off, you're already a winner.

EIGHT

"BURNING UP"

THE SYNDROME

WOULDN'T IT BE GREAT if there was a pill that could make your insulin 25 percent more effective *and* help keep your blood fats under control? Although that magic pill doesn't exist, there is something just as good: exercise. Regular aerobic exercise helps control excess insulin in the blood, as well as other manifestations of Syndrome X.

Whether in the form of walking, running, dancing, cycling, sports or any other activity that gets our blood flowing more rapidly and our breath coming harder, aerobic exercise can help control the overproduction of insulin. Aerobic activity combats the manifestations of Syndrome X by increasing insulin sensitivity and increasing glucose utilization during exercise, thereby reducing the amount of insulin your body must produce to get glucose into the cells.

Exercise studies conducted in the early 1970s showed that physically active middle-aged men had substantially lower insulin levels after an overnight fast, and released less insulin in response to a rise in blood glucose. This was because they needed less insulin to escort glucose into their cells than did their less active counterparts. In other words, they were more insulin sensitive. Further studies showed that increasing one's level of physical fitness could increase the efficiency with which glucose moved into the cells by as much as 25 percent. In brief, when you're physically fit, you need less insulin, and if you're not fit, getting into shape can dramatically reduce your insulin needs. How does simple exercise make such a big difference?

- Muscle cells don't need insulin's help to take in glucose during exercise. Muscle contractions, those repeated squeezing and relaxing motions, encourage glucose to flow into the muscle cells. This means that the pancreas won't have to pump out extra insulin in order to combat insulin resistance. Both glucose and insulin levels decrease when you exercise, and these new, healthier levels stay with you for some time even after you've finished exercising.
- The benefits of exercise are not limited to the actual act of exercising. Exercise training increases the number of GLUT 4 transporters inside your muscle and fat cells. (When insulin binds to its specific receptors on the cell membranes, the GLUT 4 transporters move to the cell walls and escort blood glucose into the cells.) The more time you spend exercising, the more of these glucose transporters your body manufactures. As a result, your body will clear glucose from your bloodstream more efficiently, and excess insulin levels will decline.

Great as exercise is, you can't just do it for a while, then drop it and expect your Syndrome X to be cured. Once you stop exercising regularly, the insulin levels you've worked so hard to drive down will shoot right back up to their old, dangerous levels. Some studies indicate that the beneficial effects of exercise only last about sixty hours; others say they may linger as long as five to seven days. Still, *any* exercise appears to be better than none at all. We know that a single exercise session can increase your insulin efficiency both during exercise and *for as much as two days afterward,* even if you are not physically fit. If you are in shape and exercise regularly, the results will be even better.

Exercise has always gone hand in hand with diet to produce maximum health benefits. Diet alone does not control insulin levels nearly as well as diet plus exercise, a team that effectively tackles the root cause of Syndrome X—insulin resistance and compensatory overproduction of insulin.

Big Returns for a Small Investment

Any increase in activity increases insulin sensitivity and helps reduce your risk of heart attack. But how much exercise do you need for optimal results? In the past, heart-health experts recommended exercising vigorously for at least 20 minutes a day, three days a week. However, further studies have led the U.S. Surgeon General and the American College of Sports Medicine to suggest 30 minutes of vigorous exercise or low-impact aerobics every day, or almost every day. But even if you are unable to exercise that much, there's still plenty you can do. Simply walking briskly for 45 minutes per day can lower your insulin resistance and aid significantly in weight loss.

A Word of Caution

Before jumping, running or diving into a new exercise program, or before increasing the amount of exercise you're currently doing, check with your physician. Have a thorough physical exam and tell your doctor which exercises you intend to do. He or she can help you develop a safe and sane program based on your age, fitness level and any medical problems, one that you can stick to without injuring yourself or "burning out." *This is especially important if you are over the age of thirty, are overweight or have any health problems. See your doctor before beginning or changing your existing exercise program if:*

- You are more than thirty years of age.
- You have been physically inactive for six or more months.
- You have a cardiovascular condition such as heart disease, high blood pressure or atherosclerosis, or have experienced dizziness, fainting, weakness or any related problems.
- You have had one or more heart attack warning signs (see below).
- You have a pulmonary condition, such as shortness of breath, asthma, emphysema, lung disease or any related problems.
- You have joint problems, such as arthritis, or related conditions that might be worsened by certain kinds of exercise.
- You have insulin-dependent diabetes. (You will need to adjust your insulin dose with exercise.)
- You have any other condition that might be aggravated by exercise.

Watch for the Signs of Heart Attack and Stroke

The fact that blood pressure rises somewhat during exercise is not a problem for most of us. But if you already have high blood pressure, even a modest increase can increase your risk of stroke, heart attack and heart failure. If you have hypertension, discuss your exercise plans with your doctor, who may suggest that you modify your activity plans, monitor your blood pressure during exercise or adjust your blood pressure medication before you begin. Start exercising slowly, increasing the intensity very gradually and only with the consent of your physician.

If you notice any of these potential warning signs of a heart attack, stop exercising immediately and get help:

- Uncomfortable pressure or pain in the chest lasting more than a few minutes
- Chest pain radiating from the chest to the shoulders, neck or arms
- Shortness of breath
- Lightheadedness, fainting, cold sweat, nausea
- Pallor or other off-color
- Dizziness
- Stomach or abdominal pain
- Difficulty breathing
- Palpitations

And if you experience any of these symptoms, which may be signs of a stroke in progress, stop exercising and get help immediately:

- Loss of sensation, weakness or paralysis in an arm, a leg or on one side of the body
- Double vision
- Partial loss of hearing or vision
- Dizziness
- Slurred speech
- Difficulty in thinking or speaking
- Loss of bladder control
- Fainting

I don't want to scare you away from exercise: most people can embark on a modest program of aerobic exercise, gradually increasing its length and intensity, without difficulty. But if you have Syndrome X or another problem that puts you at risk, it's better to be safe than sorry. See your doctor before beginning a new exercise program, or changing your current one. Start slowly, carefully increase your activity level under your physician's guidance, and watch for any signs of trouble.

Start Smart

We all know of at least one brave weekend athlete who tries to make up for six sedentary days by running 15 miles on Saturday. And we've all probably met an overzealous beginner whose first workout session lasted three hours. What happens? The weekend athlete develops an injury that leaves him sidelined for several weeks, while the neophyte exerciser gets so sore from her workout that she never wants to exercise again!

Clearly, the problem for both lies in the approach, not the exercises. Nearly everyone can avoid serious injury and/or burnout by following a few simple rules:

- Always warm up. You should do at least five, preferably ten minutes of warm-up exercises (described at the end of this chapter) to get your blood flowing and your muscles ready to contract and stretch.
- If you haven't exercised for a while, make sure your exercise routine is fairly easy—nothing too strenuous or challenging to begin with.
- Keep it short. Thirty minutes is plenty when you're just starting.
- End your exercise session with at least five minutes of cooldown exercises and stretching. The latter part of your session is the perfect time to work on your flexibility because your warmed-up muscles will stretch more easily. Stretching helps ease workout-related stiffness and sore muscles, and can also prevent future injuries.

Finding the Time

One day, out of the blue, a very busy doctor and friend of mine named Jim was struck by a heart attack. As Jim slowly and painstakingly rebuilt his health, he told me what his illness had taught him. "You've got to figure out what's most important," he said, "and allocate your time accordingly. We usually spend way too much time on the unimportant things, while neglecting the things that are really meaningful." Getting and staying healthy leapt to the top of Jim's priority list. Now, no matter how busy he is, Jim jogs, cycles or works out at the gym every single day.

You don't have to wait for a health crisis to teach you what Jim learned. Make exercise a priority; put it at the top of every day's "To Do" list, and find a way to fit it in. Believe it or not, there is *always* enough time to exercise, once you've decided it's really important. It will help if you remember that every exercise session doesn't have to be a "formal" one, that there are many ways to add "free" exercise to a busy schedule. If you are not yet exercising:

■ *Take exercise breaks at work.* Take time during the work day for a walk or calisthenics. At least 30 minutes is ideal, but if you don't have time for a long walk during your lunch hour, for example, take two shorter walks during your morning and afternoon breaks. Any exercise is better than none, and you may find that brief but brisk walks or exercise sessions reduce your stress substantially and increase your effectiveness on the job.

■ *Don't drive.* Walk or bicycle to work, to the store, to a friend's house or other places, instead of driving.

■ *Combine exercise with TV.* Can't miss the news or the soaps? Work out on a stationary bicycle or treadmill while you're watching, or do your exercise routine on a mat in front of the TV.

■ *Exercise first thing in the morning.* If you tend to peter out at the end of the day and find a million excuses not to exercise, try to get up a little earlier and get your exercise in first thing in the morning. You'll have fewer distractions and may find it easier to stick to your schedule.

Here are some more ideas:

■ Use the stairs instead of the elevator.
■ Mow your own lawn.
■ Wash your own car.
■ Walk the dog.

- Park farther away in the parking lot and walk in.
- Get off a stop early when taking rapid transit and walk the rest of the way.
- Go dancing rather than watching TV or going to the movies.
- Put away your remote control and get up to change TV channels yourself.
- Go bowling.
- Take a stroll through the park or a walk on the beach with a friend instead of meeting for coffee.

Warming Up

Be sure to warm up your muscles before using them for strenuous exercise. Muscles are a bit like your car; you need to get the motor humming and the oil circulating before putting it in gear. Exercising too hard and fast while the muscles are still cold can cause excessive stiffness, soreness, muscle strains or sprains, and/or torn ligaments.

Good warm-ups include jumping jacks, slow and gentle jogging in place, easy push-ups, rope jumping or any other mild aerobic activity that gets the blood pumping and the heart beating harder and faster. Because the muscles are not yet warm, it's best *not* to perform big stretches during the warm-up period. Moderate stretching, such as reaching your arms toward the ceiling or bending over to touch your toes, is fine at this point. But save the big stretches (i.e., the splits) until the body is thoroughly warmed. (It's safest if you wait until you've broken a sweat.)

Making Sure It's Aerobic

Although warming up and stretching are vital, the major portion of your exercise program should be devoted to aerobic exercise, activities that make your heart beat more rapidly and your breath come faster. Jogging, jumping rope, fast walking, dancing and swimming all qualify as aerobic exercise if done vigorously and continuously. Strolling at a moderate pace, gliding on a bicycle or slow dancing don't count as aerobic exercise because they aren't vigorous enough to make your heart beat continuously at a higher rate for 30 minutes.

It takes aerobic exercise to improve the health of your cardiovascular system. ("Aerobic" means "with oxygen," and aerobic exercise is defined as movement that uses oxygen to produce energy over a sustained period of time.) How do you know if you're exercising hard enough to gain aerobic benefits? Use the American College of Sports Medicine's guidelines for target heart range to see if you're exercising vigorously enough. If the activity keeps your heart continuously beating in the target range for 30 minutes, it's aerobic. Here's how you figure your range:

1. Subtract your age from 220.
2. Multiply the answer from Step 1 by 0.6 to find the lower end of your target heart rate zone.
3. Multiply the answer from Step 1 by 0.8 to find the upper end of your target heart rate zone.

Here's an example for a forty-five-year-old.

1. Subtract your age from 220: 220 − 45 = 175
2. Multiply the answer from Step 1 by 0.6 to find the lower end of your target heart rate zone: 175 × 0.6 = 105
3. Multiply the answer from Step 1 by 0.8 to find the upper end of your target heart rate zone: 175 × 0.8 = 140

To gain aerobic benefits, this forty-five-year-old person would have to move vigorously enough to keep his or her heart beating between 105 and 140 beats per minute for 30 minutes.

How do you know if you're within your target heart rate zone? All you need is a clock or stopwatch with a second hand. Find your pulse by placing your index and second fingers on the inside of your opposite wrist, on the far side of the most prominent tendon. Count the number of beats for 15 seconds and multiply by 4 to find your heart rate.

Remember, these recommendations for length and intensity of exercise are goals, not hard-and-fast rules. If you haven't exercised in a while or have health problems, you may need to start with slow, gentle exercise. That's fine. Do what you can without undue strain. If you can exercise for only 5 or 10 minutes a day the first week, fine. You've started. Keep building until you can do at least 30 minutes of aerobic activity per day. The main thing is to do *something*. You can—and will—improve with time.

Dressing for the Occasion

What you wear while you exercise matters more than you might think. Not only do your clothes and shoes have a substantial effect on your comfort, they can help prevent injury. For example, wearing properly fitting, shock-absorbing running shoes can help you prevent shin splints and joint injuries, especially when you're running on paved surfaces. Knee and elbow pads can help prevent bruises and abrasions should you fall when rollerblading, while helmets guard against head injuries. And lightweight cotton clothing that wicks moisture away from the skin can help prevent heat exhaustion.

Besides the obvious safety and comfort functions, clothes can give you a psychological lift and make exercise more fun. So go ahead, buy that wild aerobics outfit or those fabulous tennis shoes that make you feel like you can run faster and jump higher. If you feel good in your clothes and good about yourself, you'll be more likely to go out and move!

Make It Fun!

If exercise is dull, you probably won't stick with it for long. So be creative when choosing your activities. When my three children were young, we used to play a rousing game of basketball before dinner. Now that they've grown up, I prefer to jog in the mornings: it fits well into my schedule and gives me time to think about my goals for the day.

One of my patients joined a weekly ballroom dance class where he and his wife have a great time twirling and whirling their way to better health. Four or five other days a week they walk briskly around the park, bicycle at a pretty good clip or rollerblade. A group of people at the office who call themselves the "Lunchtime Walking Brigade" bring tennis shoes and sweats to work, change at lunch time and take brisk 45-minute walks through the nearby neighborhoods. A friend of mine bicycles to work two days a week, ten miles each way. Another walks to work, racking up a total of six miles round trip daily. One woman I know goes to ballet class two evenings a week and jazz dancing on Saturday mornings. She swears that dance has kept the years at bay and, indeed, she does have the body of a much younger woman.

The best exercise advice I can give you is this: find activities that you enjoy and that fit well into your daily schedule. Then you'll be much more likely to exercise on a regular basis. Here are some of the more popular aerobic activities:

- *Brisk walking*—A popular, inexpensive form of exercise. All you need is a good pair of supportive shoes and some loose-fitting clothes appropriate to the season. You can do it just about anywhere, and it puts much less strain on the bones, joints and ligaments than intense running. You can also suit your current level of conditioning by pacing yourself, choosing any speed from strolling to race-walking.
- *Jogging/running*—This is another simple, inexpensive way to get into shape. Remember, however, that too much "pavement pounding" can cause joint troubles. To avoid overstressing the joints, many people jog or run only one or two days a week, then swim or bicycle the other days.
- *Cycling*—This excellent aerobic activity is easy on the joints because you're not pounding your feet on the ground. It also helps tone and strengthen your leg muscles. If you're not the outdoor type, you can bicycle indoors on a stationary bike, reading or watching TV as you pedal away.
- *Swimming*—Swimming uses all of the major muscle groups, and is well suited to people who have joint problems because the water supports the body while simultaneously providing resistance. You can get plenty of exercise without putting wear and tear on your joints.
- *Aerobics*—If you enjoy moving to music, aerobics classes may be for you. You might have to shop around a bit for an appropriate activity level and teaching style, but the effort will be worth it. Make sure you have a good pair of supportive shoes and comfortable clothes. If you have joint problems, look for a "low-impact" class which will limit jumping, pounding and other movements that overload the joints.
- *Cross-country skiing*—Whether you live in snow country or prefer to "ski" on a machine indoors, cross-country skiing is one of the very best overall conditioning exercises. It uses many muscle groups but puts very little stress on your knees because your feet slide rather than pound on the ground.
- *Hiking*—Hiking, particularly uphill, can provide an inexpensive, hefty and exhilarating workout. If you love being out-

doors among beautiful scenery, you'll probably find that 30 minutes just isn't long enough! A good pair of all-weather hiking boots that support the ankles and have lug soles to prevent slippage is a must, as is a thick pair of socks to protect your feet from abrasion and blisters.

■ *Rowing*—Whether on a lake or using a machine that's firmly planted on dry land, rowing can give you a tremendous aerobic workout while helping to build your arm and back muscles.

As you put together your exercise program, pick and choose from among these or any other exercises that interest you. Remember: the best exercise isn't necessarily the one providing the greatest overall strength and flexibility, the most comprehensive cardiovascular workout or the most fabulous body sculpting. It's the one that you'll actually *do!* And that depends entirely on your interests, which activities "feel right" to your body, and your level of commitment and motivation. You don't have to—and you shouldn't—stick to just one kind of activity. Variety is the spice of life, especially where exercise is concerned. Do you like to dance? Swing dancing is a great form of aerobic exercise. How about kayaking on a river or in the ocean? If it sounds good, give it a try. Keep in mind that if you're having fun, you're far more likely to keep exercising!

STRETCHING

Just five minutes of stretching at the end of your exercise session will help prevent injury, burn calories, maintain flexibility and even reduce the amount of muscle soreness you'll feel tomorrow! And although 5 minutes is good, 10, 15 or 20 minutes is even better.

The most important things to remember about stretching are:

■ *Never stretch a cold muscle.* Always make sure you've broken a sweat before doing any big stretches.

■ *Stretch to the point where you feel resistance, but no pain.* If it hurts, you're probably stretching too far. Ease off.

■ *Stretch to your maximum position, then hold it for 15 seconds.* Static stretching (staying in one position) is the healthiest and safest way to stretch. Stretch as far as you can without feeling pain, and hold that position without moving for at least 15 seconds. Then relax and slowly ease off.

- *Don't "bounce" while you stretch.* Stretching and then releasing a muscle in several quick bursts invites strain and sprain. Muscles should always be stretched slowly and carefully.
- *Make sure you're performing the stretch properly.* You can strain or even tear muscles and ligaments by stretching incorrectly. It's best to begin stretching under the supervision of a qualified instructor who can show you the proper methods. Once you've learned the basics, you can stretch on your own.

Stretches for Anyone

Just about anyone can do these simple stretches, which improve flexibility, encourage relaxation and make you feel great all over!

Lengthening Stretch. Stand with feet together, arms extended above your head, palms facing each other and about 18 inches apart. Reach the right arm up toward the ceiling, feeling the stretch in your right side. Release slightly. Then reach the left arm up, feeling the stretch in your left side. Release. Repeat, alternating sides for 8 counts. Then stand with the feet parallel and about 18 inches apart. Repeat arm stretches for 8 counts. Go back to feet together and stretch 8 counts; then another 8 counts with feet parallel.

Side-to-Side Stretch. Stand with feet parallel and 18 inches apart. Place left hand on your left hip. Extend right arm over your head and bend sideways toward the left, with head facing front. You'll feel the stretch all along your right side. Return to starting position. Repeat on the right side, feeling the stretch in your left side. Take at least 4 slow counts to get to your maximum position (bent sideways), hold 4 counts, then take 4 counts to return to starting position. Do at least 4 of these stretches on each side.

Calf Stretch. Face a wall, with feet parallel and about 10 inches apart, and toes 24 inches from the wall's surface. Keeping feet parallel and apart, slide the right foot back about 12 inches, so that the left foot is now forward. Lean forward and place your palms against the wall, supporting your body at a 45-degree angle and bending your left knee while keeping your right leg as straight as possible. You should feel a nice stretch in the right calf, especially if you keep your right heel in contact with the floor. Reverse positions to stretch the left calf. For an Achilles tendon stretch, repeat the calf stretch but bend both knees during the stretch. Be very careful when stretching the Achilles tendon, as it can be injured easily.

Thigh Stretch. Stand facing a wall, with your feet slightly apart. Place your right palm against the wall for support, then bend your left knee and bring your left foot up toward your buttocks. Grasp your ankle with your left hand and pull your foot gently up toward your buttocks. The thigh should be in its usual position, in line with the torso. Hold this stretch to a count of 20, release and bring your foot back down to the ground. Repeat, stretching the right thigh. Alternate legs, repeating at least two more times.

Arm Rotation. Extend your arms to the side at shoulder level. Make fists, with palms up. Rotate your arms backward 8 times in large circles, then gradually increase the tension during the next 8 counts, making smaller circles. Relax, then repeat, rotating arms forward.

These are just a few of the numerous stretches that almost everyone can do. A fitness instructor or exercise physiologist can show you many more good ones.

EXERCISES FOR THOSE WITH SPECIAL PROBLEMS

Don't despair if you have heart disease, arthritis, osteoporosis or some other ailment that prevents you from performing vigorous exercises. You can still perform aerobic exercises, become stronger and more flexible. Low-impact exercises such as walking and swimming can go a long way toward increasing fitness if done regularly and for sustained periods of time. Even gardening and housework are helpful. The point is to get moving and keep moving, no matter what your current fitness level. As long as you stick to a regular program, gradually increasing the intensity and duration of activity, you're bound to improve your overall fitness.

Seated Exercises

If you have heart disease and need to take it easy while exercising, doing seated exercises can be just the ticket, improving fitness, flexibility and strength. Seated exercises are also recommended for those who have joint or bone problems, or lack the strength and/or balance to do standing exercises.

Here are just a few of the many seated exercises you can try. Find a comfortable, straight-backed chair without arms that sits securely on the floor and try any or all of the following:

Seated Warm-Up

Seated Jumping Jacks. Place feet together flat on the floor, arms hanging down at your sides. Keeping your arms straight, swing them out to the side and over your head, touching the backs of your hands together. At the same time, move your feet as far apart as is comfortable. Bring your arms and feet back to their original position. Repeat 10 to 25 times.

Seated Marching. Sit up straight with your feet flat on the floor and slightly apart. Lift your right foot 3 to 8 inches off the floor (but not more than is comfortable). Then lower it and raise the left foot. "March" in this manner for one to two minutes.

Seated Swimming. Pretend you are doing the crawl stroke, moving your arms alternately through the air for at least one minute (longer, if you like). To avoid joint problems, keep your arms shoulder width apart, making sure you do not cross your hands in front of you as you stroke. Repeat with one or more minutes of backstroke, then add the breaststroke.

Seated Aerobic Exercises

Seated Running. After you've completed seated marching, pick up the pace and move into seated running for one to two minutes. Be careful not to slam your feet against the floor.

Seated Fencing. With both feet flat on the floor and your left foot slid forward several inches, place your right fist on the center of your chest, elbow parallel to the floor. Exhaling, thrust your tensed right arm forward in a stabbing motion. As you inhale, bring your fist back to your chest. Repeat the movement 10 times; then slide your left foot back and your right foot forward and place your left fist on the center of your chest. Thrust out the left arm 10 times. "Fence" left and right for one to two minutes.

Seated Single Arm Extensions. Begin with your arms at your sides. Inhale deeply. Tense and straighten your right arm like a sword, lifting it up in front of you and extending it over your head. Exhale as you bring your arm down to starting position, then relax. Repeat exercise with your left arm, alternating arms for one to three minutes. For greater effect, use light weights.

Seated Leg Swings. Grasp the edge of the chair seat for balance and place your feet close together, lifting them slightly off the floor. Swing your feet 6 or 8 inches to the left and tap your toes on the floor. Then lift your feet and swing them to the right and tap the floor. Repeat for one to two minutes.

Stationary Cycling. Practically every gym and fitness club has stationary bicycles that can give you a great aerobic workout. You can also purchase mechanical or electronic models for your home.

Stationary Arm Pedaling. Although not as popular as stationary bicycles, some clubs and gyms have "arm pedaling" machines. They're very similar to stationary bicycles but the pedals are in front of you, at approximately shoulder height, and you work them with your arms, not your legs.

Seated Stretches and Cooldown

Seated Neck Rotations. Drop your head to the right, your right ear attempting to touch your right shoulder. Place your right hand on the left side of your head, just above the left ear, and put your left hand on your left shoulder. Gently press with both hands, stretching the left side of your neck. Release. Rotate your head toward the back, chin pointing toward the ceiling, to stretch the front of the neck. Rotate the head toward the left and stretch the right side of the neck in the same manner that the left side of neck was stretched. Release. Then interlace the fingers, place them on the back of the head and pull the head forward, attempting to place the chin on the chest. Release. Repeat the entire sequence.

Seated Shoulder Rotation. Sitting up straight with your fingertips touching your shoulders, rotate both shoulders up, back, down and forward again, forming large circles. Do 4 "back" circles, then rotate 4 times forward.

Seated Side Stretches. Start with your right arm relaxed and hanging down by your side. Your left arm is bent, hand resting on your hip. Extend your right arm straight up above your head. Lean to the left as far as is comfortable, keeping right arm extended and nearly in contact with your right ear. Then straighten up, and slowly return your right arm to your side. Repeat the exercise on the left side. Do at least 5 sets.

Seated Knee Pulls. Grasp one knee with both hands and slowly pull toward your chest, keeping your back straight. Hold for five seconds, then release. Repeat with other knee. Do 4 on each side.

Seated Calf Stretch. Sit up straight with both feet on the floor. Lift your right leg up with the knee bent, then straighten it out in front of you as far as possible. You should feel a tightening in the front of your thigh, along with a stretch in your calf and the back of your thigh. Bend the knee and bring your foot to the floor. Repeat 6 times on the right and 6 times on the left.

Seated Ankle Stretch. With your feet flat on the floor, lift your right heel while keeping the ball of the foot in contact with the floor. Bring heel down, then raise the toes and the arch, while keeping heel in contact with the floor. Repeat 8 times, alternately lifting heel and toes. Then repeat with left foot.

Seated Ankle Rotation. Lift your right foot off the floor 3 inches. With gentle tension, rotate your foot in small circles, 8 times to the right and 8 times to the left. It's as if you're drawing an imaginary circle in the air with your big toe. Relax. Repeat the exercise with the left foot.

Seated Relaxation. Inhale deeply and tense your toes. Without releasing the tension, tense your feet, then your ankles, calves, thighs and so on all the way up to your face. When you reach the top of your head, hold the tension throughout your body and feel the vibration. Then release the tension, one body part at a time, beginning with the face and continuing down to the toes. Relax completely. Repeat 4 times.

Like Money in the Bank

Exercise pays big dividends; it's well worth whatever time or money you invest. You can do a great deal to control or even eliminate disease, including Syndrome X, just by putting on those tennis shoes and going for a brisk walk! And in the process, you'll strengthen your cardiovascular system, improve your lung capacity, lower your body fat, lower your blood fats and even improve your looks. So what are you waiting for? Get moving—you have everything to gain!

DRINKING, SMOKING
AND SYNDROME X

A SUCCESSFUL COMPUTER SALESMAN, Charles was convinced that he could overcome just about any problem facing him. So when his doctor told him that the results of his annual examination were disturbing, forty-two-year-old Charles was not alarmed.

"I thought the doc was overreacting when he told me that my blood pressure, which had always been in the high-normal range, was elevated, that my triglycerides had gone up from 180 to 275 and that my HDL had dropped to 40. That was the lowest it had ever been. The doc wanted to give me one drug for my blood pressure and one for my triglycerides, but I wasn't keen on taking medicines. I grew up thinking that the fewer drugs you take, the better. I still believe that.

"Instead of drugs, I asked if there was anything else I could do. And I promised to follow any advice he gave me. He said I was overweight and that losing fifteen pounds would help lower both my triglycerides and my blood pressure. And even if losing weight didn't solve all my problems, he said it would certainly improve things."

Charles left his doctor's office with a low-calorie diet that the nurse had given him. When he examined the diet at home that night, he thought it looked pretty easy to follow, not much different from what he thought he was already eating. He felt confident that he could lose the extra weight and get his blood pressure and triglycerides back in line.

For the next several months Charles worked hard at sticking to his diet, even though his job as a salesman dictated that he entertain clients and eat out often. But to his great surprise and dismay, his weight hardly budged. At the rate he was going, it would take months to lose those fifteen pounds.

"I used to make fun of my friends who said they couldn't lose weight," said Charles. "I'd always sort of laughed to myself when they said they gained weight no matter how little they ate. But suddenly it didn't seem so funny, now that my own excess weight wasn't coming off. I knew I was following the diet pretty much to the letter, so I figured I must have some sort of metabolic problem. I was too embarrassed to go back to my doctor weighing what I did, so I made an appointment with Dr. Reaven at the Stanford University Clinic."

During the examination, a chagrined Charles complained that he couldn't seem to lose weight, no mater how carefully he dieted. Repeat laboratory studies were almost identical to his earlier ones: his blood pressure and triglycerides were still too high, and his HDL too low. All that work, and nothing had really changed!

As Charles and I reviewed his lifestyle, the key to his problem suddenly became obvious. This salesman regularly entertained clients at meals, receptions and parties. As Charles put it, "There's usually some wine with dinner, or a couple beers if we go to a ball game or golfing. But I make it a point not to drink too much, so I never thought anything of it. Then the doctor told me how many calories there are in alcohol. I was stunned! Between my business lunches and dinner meetings with clients, and a little social drinking on the weekend, I was losing all the progress I made on my diet."

Alcohol does indeed contain calories. For example, a bottle of beer, a gin martini or two small glasses of wine all have approximately 150 calories. Drink two glasses of wine at dinner and you add 150 calories to your daily intake. Sip two beers at the football game and you've added 300 calories. It sneaks up on you. And remember, a calorie is a calorie, it doesn't matter where it comes from. A calorie from a vodka martini provides the same amount of energy as a calorie from butter, and can make you gain the same amount of weight. If you're already consuming enough calories from food to meet your daily energy needs, these extra calories from alcohol can quickly add up to weight gain. If you're trying to follow a weight-loss diet, they can sabotage even the most valiant efforts.

Remember, too, that when alcohol is metabolized, the body converts it to fatty acids, which can stimulate your liver to make more triglycerides. Charles's business and social drinking prevented him from losing weight *and* kept his triglyceride levels up.

ALCOHOL AND SYNDROME X

It's difficult to separate scientific data from philosophic beliefs about alcohol. Perhaps there are only two unequivocal facts. One is that excessive consumption of alcohol—more than two to three drinks per day—is harmful to your health, whether you have Syndrome X or not.

What Is a "Drink"?

A "drink" (or one serving of an alcoholic beverage) is defined by the amount of alcohol in the fluid, not the amount of fluid itself. Although their sizes may vary considerably, each of the following contains approximately the same amount of alcohol, making each a single drink of an alcoholic beverage:

- 12 ounces of beer, or about a mug's worth
- 5 ounces of wine, which is about what you get in one glass
- 1¼–1½ ounces of liquor, spirits or the "hard stuff," which is about what you get in a shot glass

---

The second unequivocal fact is that although there appear to be some health benefits associated with moderate alcohol consumption (one to three drinks per day), no one should begin drinking just to get these benefits. Research shows that people consuming one to three drinks per day have less coronary heart disease than nondrinkers, but there is no hard-and-fast evidence demonstrating that nondrinkers will enjoy significant health benefits if they start drinking. You can gain these health-boosting effects just by changing your diet and exercise regimen, while avoiding the risks associated with excessive drinking.

Coronary Heart Disease Risk and Alcohol Consumption

Several epidemiological studies looking at large population groups have found that the risk of heart disease is inversely proportional to

HDL "good" cholesterol concentration. In other words, the higher your HDL cholesterol, the lower your risk of heart disease. These same studies found a strong relationship between alcohol consumption and HDL cholesterol concentration: up to a moderate intake of one to three drinks per day, more alcohol equals more HDL.

Remember, however, that showing that moderate drinkers tend to have higher HDL levels does not prove that it's the drinking that elevates HDL. There may be other factors we're unaware of. As yet, we cannot conclusively prove that moderate drinkers have a reduced risk of heart disease *because* the alcohol they drink is pushing up their HDL cholesterol.

Alcohol and Insulin

About the same time we realized that HDL cholesterol concentrations were higher in moderate drinkers, totally different lines of scientific investigation revealed a very close relationship between the degree of insulin resistance, hyperinsulinemia and HDL cholesterol levels.

Noting that there seemed to be some link between moderate alcohol consumption, higher levels of HDL and protection against heart disease, and knowing that people with insulin resistance and compensatory hyperinsulinemia tended to have lower HDL, we wondered if insulin resistance might explain why moderate drinking seemed to protect against heart disease. Could it be that moderate drinkers were more insulin sensitive than nondrinkers? If that were so, it would help to explain why they had higher HDL cholesterol levels and less risk of heart attack.

As we were performing studies to test this hypothesis, a paper supporting our theory was published in the United Kingdom. Studies of large population groups had shown that insulin levels were indeed lower, and HDL cholesterol levels higher, in those who enjoyed one to three drinks per day.

We were quite pleased when we saw these results, for they substantiated our own thoughts. Shortly thereafter, we completed our study[1] in normal volunteers, and for the first time published evidence that moderate drinkers were more insulin sensitive and had lower insulin levels and higher HDL cholesterol levels than nondrinkers.

[1] F. Facchini, Y. D. Chen, and G. R. Reaven. "Light-to-moderate alcohol intake is associated with enhanced insulin sensitivity." *Diabetes Care* (1994) 17(2):115–118.

Insulin, Heart Health and Alcohol

To verify the link between insulin sensitivity and light-to-moderate alcohol consumption, my colleagues and I enlisted forty healthy volunteers as subjects for our study performed at Stanford University. The twenty men and twenty women participating in this case-controlled study were divided into two groups: nondrinkers and light-to-moderate drinkers. The participants in each group were carefully matched by age, sex and degrees of obesity and physical activity. We took various measurements of their insulin and glucose levels—before and after consuming a sugary drink, etc. The results were quite clear: volunteers who consumed light-to-moderate amounts of alcohol were more insulin sensitive. They had lower blood sugar and lower insulin levels after drinking a sugary fluid, and higher HDL cholesterol levels.

It seems clear that people who consume light-to-moderate amounts of alcohol are more insulin sensitive and have lower insulin levels and higher HDL cholesterol levels than those who do not. This should decrease their chances of suffering heart attacks. But don't start drinking to protect your heart. Remember, there is absolutely no evidence showing that insulin sensitivity will improve when a nondrinker begins quaffing the brews. Moderate alcohol consumption is absolutely not a recommended treatment for Syndrome X.

When Is Alcohol Harmful?

We know that excessive alcohol consumption can trigger serious diseases involving essentially every body system. But is moderate drinking also harmful? Can it exacerbate Syndrome X? In some cases the answer may be yes, especially where alcohol's effect on triglycerides is concerned.

Elevated triglyceride concentration is the most common abnormality in Syndrome X. Since alcohol consumption can increase triglycerides, we might argue that people with the syndrome should abstain. Although this is certainly a simple solution, it's a bit rigid.

The higher the triglyceride concentrations and the more alcohol one consumes, the greater the increase in plasma triglycerides. But unless your blood fat levels are quite high (more than 250 mg/dl), having one to three drinks per day is probably not going to adversely affect the syndrome's manifestations. Here are general guidelines for those with Syndrome X:

1. If your blood triglyceride level is less than 150 mg/dl and you are a moderate drinker, there is no reason to change your drinking habits.
2. If your triglyceride level is greater than 250 mg/dl, stop drinking and see if it comes down. You should do this whether or not you make any other lifestyles changes to combat Syndrome X.
3. If your triglyceride levels remain between 150 and 250 mg/dl even after making the lifestyle improvements described in this book, it would be reasonable to decrease your alcoholic intake to see if your levels fall. If so, keep cutting back on your alcohol consumption until your triglyceride level drops to less than 150 mg/dl. If you gain nothing by decreasing your current level of alcohol intake, it is obvious that alcohol is not contributing to your hypertriglyceridemia.

Absent very high triglyceride levels or a special sensitivity to the effects of alcohol on triglyceride metabolism, there's no reason for those with Syndrome X to give up moderate drinking.

Does It Matter What You Drink?

A great deal has been written about the health-related benefits of one alcoholic beverage over another. Most of it is pure myth. It makes for great cocktail conversation, but is not backed by the scientific evidence. For example, many people believe that red wine is more heart protective than other alcoholic beverages. Although the theories offered to support this argument are intriguing, there is simply no evidence that red wine protects the heart more than white wine, beer or spirits. As long as the alcoholic content is similar, all drinks seem equally good for the heart *when taken in moderation*.

Remember: while heart disease is lower in moderate drinkers than in nondrinkers, there is no evidence that moderate drinking can overcome the bad effects of an unhealthy diet, a sedentary lifestyle or other poor health habits. There is, on the other hand, evidence to suggest that some of alcohol's beneficial effects on the heart may stem from its interaction with certain Syndrome X factors. The wisest approach is to drink only in moderation, and if you don't already drink, don't start.

SMOKING AND SYNDROME X

There is absolutely no doubt that the prevalence of coronary heart disease, lung cancer, chronic respiratory disease and other ailments would fall dramatically if everyone quit smoking. The scientific evidence showing this to be true is unequivocal. What we don't know is how and why this is true.

That cigarette smoking is a major risk factor for coronary heart disease has been proven by numerous epidemiological and other studies. But scientists are still struggling to understand the specific link between smoking and heart disease. It may be that nicotine or one of the many other chemicals in cigarettes accelerates cellular processes that lead to fat deposits in the coronary arteries. Components in the cigarette smoke itself may encourage atherosclerosis developing in coronary arteries.

Recently published research has provided new insight into why smoking is such a powerful risk factor for coronary heart disease, whether or not you have Syndrome X. It's also clear that smokers with Syndrome X are at even greater than average risk of being slammed with heart attacks.

What's in a Cigarette?

The complete list of ingredients is too long to print here. Just the tar in cigarette smoke contains thousands of different chemical substances, some forty of which are known to be carcinogenic. As you puff you'll inhale acetylene (torch fuel), ammonia, benzene, carbon monoxide (a poisonous gas), cyanide, formaldehyde, methanol (wood alcohol), nitrogen oxide (a poisonous gas) and, of course, nicotine.

The list of diseases definitely linked to smoking is equally impressive, in a negative sense. These ailments include numerous forms of cancer, heart disease, emphysema, chronic bronchitis, stillbirth and spontaneous abortion. Smoking also causes fatigue and interferes with the senses of smell and taste.

The first of these newer studies delving into the cigarette smoking/heart disease connection came out of my own laboratory at Stanford University in 1992.[2] Several large epidemiological studies had already made it clear that smokers, as a group, have higher blood triglyceride and lower HDL "good" cholesterol levels than do nonsmokers. Knowing this, my research group and I put together a hypothesis linking cigarette smoking and heart disease to Syndrome X. Here's how our reasoning went:

- Insulin resistance and compensatory hyperinsulinemia cause triglycerides to rise and HDL cholesterol levels to fall.
- Smokers have higher triglyceride and lower HDL levels.
- There appears to be a link between cigarette smoking and heart disease.
- Therefore, at least some portion of the bad effects of smoking on heart disease is due to changes in the triglyceride and HDL cholesterol concentrations in smokers.
- In other words, smokers might have these Syndrome X abnormalities.

To test our hypotheses, we divided forty healthy volunteers in their late thirties and early forties into two equal groups, one composed of nonsmokers and the other of smokers who had smoked at least one pack of cigarettes daily for a minimum of six years. The smokers were more insulin resistant than the nonsmokers. We then measured their plasma glucose and insulin concentrations before and after giving them a 75 gram glucose drink.

Blood sugar levels were just a little higher in the smokers than in the nonsmokers in response to the glucose challenge. Insulin concentrations, however, rose much higher in the smokers. Their pancreases were able to secrete enough insulin to overcome their insulin resistance and prevent their glucose levels from going too high, but they paid a price for this insulin resistance and compensatory hyperinsulinemia: almost a doubling of triglyceride-rich VLDL and a 30 percent fall in HDL cholesterol. These are the classic changes seen in Syndrome X.

These results once again showed that triglyceride levels were higher and HDL cholesterol levels lower in smokers compared with

[2] F. S. Facchini, C. B. Hollenbeck, J. Jeppesen, Y. D. Chen, G. R. Reaven. "Insulin resistance and cigarette smoking." *Lancet* (1992) 339:1128–1130.

nonsmokers. The data also confirmed our hypothesis that smokers are significantly more insulin resistant and have higher plasma insulin levels than do nonsmokers. In other words, smokers were more likely to develop the syndrome and/or to be hit harder.

Our study definitely linked cigarette smoking to Syndrome X. Subsequent studies performed in several European countries have confirmed these results. In particular, Swedish studies have greatly added to our understanding of the link between smoking and insulin metabolism. For instance, we now know that chronic smokers are not just more insulin resistant during the few minutes it takes them to smoke a cigarette. As long as they keep smoking, chronic smokers remain insulin resistant *between* cigarettes as well. And the more cigarettes smoked, the greater the effect on insulin resistance. Equally important, we now know that insulin resistance improves when smokers stop smoking.

No one should smoke. It is bad for your health whether you have Syndrome X or not. Smoking is associated with insulin resistance, elevated triglyceride and lower HDL "good" cholesterol. Smokers have an even greater risk of developing *all* of the manifestations of Syndrome X than do insulin-resistant nonsmokers. And if you are already at risk of developing Syndrome X, smoking will increase the likelihood that it will strike. There could hardly be a stronger incentive to stop smoking—now!

Smoking Cessation

Quitting may be tough, but it is well worth the effort. Within a year after you take your last puff, lung damage begins to repair itself, and by year five, your risk of dying from lung cancer is cut almost in half. Fifteen years after you puff your last, you are no more likely to develop coronary heart disease than nonsmokers, and only slightly more likely to die of lung cancer. When you quit, your risk of developing cancer of the lung, mouth, esophagus, pancreas, bladder or cervix drops significantly.

There is no perfect one-size-fits-all method of quitting. However, there are two things that all successful approaches have in common: commitment and understanding. You must make a firm commitment to quitting, and set a firm stopping date. And you have to understand that it won't be easy, because your mind and body have come to rely on tobacco. For the first three to five days after stopping, you may experience unpleasant physical withdrawal symptoms. Even as the physical symptoms subside, you may still have a strong desire for a cigarette, especially at specific times of the day, or when you're doing certain things. You may have the urge to "light up" after a meal, or when you settle into the driver's seat of your car. The urge to smoke may continue for months or years; desires may come and go. Fortunately, the urges grow weaker and your will stronger as time passes.

The first week is likely to be the most difficult, which is why many people relapse and go back to smoking in those first seven days. Often they do so because their addiction is strong, or they haven't developed the social and family support they need. And once past that first week, they're still not out of the woods. Many will surrender to their urges during the first three months, usually because they haven't replaced their old habits with new nonsmoking ones. Here are some tips that can help you kick the habit once and for all, regardless of which program you use.

- *Know why you're quitting.* Draw up a list of reasons why you want to quit. Review that list several times a day before you quit, while you're quitting, and every day afterwards.
- *Pick a quitting date.* Pick a date, one that will come fairly soon. Selecting a date helps you firm up your commitment.
- *Tell everyone that you're quitting.* Tell your family, friends and colleagues that you plan to quit on such and such day. Explain why and ask for their support. If a family member or close friend is also a smoker, ask him or her to quit with you.
- *Prepare to quit.* There are many things you can do to ease the transition to nonsmoker. Gradually taper off, smoking fewer cigarettes a day. Smoke the same number of cigarettes, but only half of each. Switch to a less appealing brand, or one with less nicotine. Keep reviewing your list of reasons to quit, reminding yourself of the great health and other benefits that await. Wash the cigarette smoke out of your clothes, and notice that they no longer stink all the time. Make smoking a little more difficult by tossing out your favorite lighters or ashtrays. Keep just one ashtray and clean it every time you use it. Buy your cigarettes by the pack instead of the carton so it becomes a drag to keep stocked up. Store your pack in an inconvenient place. Anything you can to do to cut back, to remind yourself of the benefits of quitting and to make it a little tougher to indulge your habit, will be helpful.

- *Take it one day at a time.* Every day, renew your commitment to quitting. Review your reasons for stopping and focus on getting through today. You can deal with tomorrow, tomorrow.
- *Make it tough to puff.* Much of smoking is ritualized behavior: you smoke when you drink a cup of coffee or go to a party because you're used to doing so. These are "trigger" activities. Make it tough to puff by taking a long walk or a shower, by swimming, mowing the lawn, washing the car, going dancing or otherwise avoiding the trigger activities. Attack the ingrained habits of smoking by planning ahead. If you used to smoke after each meal, get up and get away from the table as soon as you finish eating. Take the ashtray out of your car if you always smoked while driving, or deliberately sit in the non-smoking section of a restaurant.
- *Beat the clock.* When you feel the urge to smoke, take out your watch and time it. You'll be surprised to see how briefly the urge remains. Knowing how short and transitory the urges are will help you resist them.
- *Never give in!* The successful quitters are the ones who refuse to give up, who never give in to the urge to light one up, or who start again when they've slipped. Keep trying! If you catch yourself saying something like "I just can't do it," say instead, "I can hang in for another few minutes until the urge has passed," or "I can do this!" Reward yourself when you safely ride out an urge. Put the money you save by not buying cigarettes toward something fun. If you do light a cigarette, don't smoke it. If you begin to smoke, stop halfway. If you finish the cigarette, don't despair. Stay focused on thoughts of the day when you'll be able to go twenty-four hours without smoking. Review your list of reasons for quitting. Imagine what it will be like to be rid of the smoker's hacking cough, to have clothes that smell fresh, to get rid of the yellow stains on your teeth and fingernails. Think how great it will feel to breathe easy and have lots of stamina.
- *Get help when you need it.* There are numerous approaches and aids to help you, including nicotine patches and gum, self-help groups, counseling, acupuncture and hypnosis. Medicines such as clonidine may help with the withdrawal symptoms.
- *Be realistic.* Quitting is not easy. Immediately after you stop, you may feel irritable, on edge, hungry or tired. You may have trouble sleeping for a while. Don't be alarmed; these are common symptoms of nicotine withdrawal. Most of the nicotine will be

cleared from your body within two to three days after you stop smoking, but your desire for nicotine may last for weeks. Many people feel hungry when they quit; others simply want to put something in their mouths. Either urge can cause you to gain weight. If you do put on a little weight, resolve to lose it once you've conquered your smoking problem. To help avoid putting it on in the first place, watch your diet carefully, keep low-calorie snacks and beverages handy, and drink a glass of water before each meal to help fill you up. If you need oral gratification, try chewing sugarless gum or munching on celery, carrots or sunflower seeds. And be sure to exercise regularly. Some people become constipated immediately after they quit. If this happens to you, add more fruits, vegetables and whole grains to your diet.

Giving up tobacco may be difficult, but it's well worth the effort whether you have Syndrome X or not. Never stop trying to quit, no matter how many times you must try before you successfully quit. This is one time when being a quitter means being a winner!

SHOULD MEDICINE

BE NECESSARY

BARBARA SIGHED DEEPLY AS she looked in the mirror. The last fifteen pounds she'd been trying to lose for almost a year clung to her middle as tenaciously as a barnacle on a ship's side. At first she had wanted to shed those pounds for vanity's sake, but now it seemed that more than her appearance was at stake. Her blood pressure was a little high at 150/90, her triglycerides had jumped to 215 and her HDL "good" cholesterol had fallen to 30. Then her total cholesterol weighed in at an alarming 240, which meant that her LDL cholesterol was elevated. Barbara's doctor sternly told her that she must lose weight. Now she felt increasingly guilty about every bite she put into her mouth and every exercise session she skipped, and increasingly alarmed about the state of her health.

Barbara came to the clinic practically in tears. "I can't seem to lose these last fifteen pounds," she wailed. "I've tried and tried, but I just can't seem to do it. And I'm terrified of having a heart attack. What should I do?"

We urged her not to despair. Although diet and exercise are important elements in the Syndrome X program, they aren't the whole answer. Even if you manage to fit into the clothes you wore back in high school, and even if you jog thirty minutes a day, four days a week, you may still have some elements of Syndrome X.

A thirty-five-year-old woman named Ladrina also wanted to lose weight, but for a different reason. Her mother, who had suffered from type 2 diabetes, had died of a heart attack just a few months earlier. Ladrina was anxious to find out if she, too, was in danger, so she had blood and glucose tolerance tests performed at the clinic. The results were unnerving, to say the least.

"My results were far from what I had hoped for," Ladrina sighed. "My total cholesterol was nice and low at 140, but my triglycerides were way too high at 225 and my HDL was only 33. I wasn't diabetic yet, but the doctor said I had impaired glucose tolerance, which could lead to diabetes. So there I was, tottering on the edges of both type 2 diabetes and a heart attack. I was sure it was only a matter of time before I had a heart attack.

"When the doctor told me to lose weight and exercise, I knew it wouldn't be easy. I had wrenched my knee when I was a kid and I had a lot of pain sometimes. So I decided to take up swimming since it wouldn't put a lot of stress on my joints. It surprised me when I really got into it. I started going three mornings a week to swim, and I did a special 'sit-down exercise program' on three other mornings. Sunday mornings I just slept in."

When Ladrina returned to her doctor three months later, she had lost eight pounds and her test results had improved. Her triglycerides had dropped from 225 to 180, and her HDL had risen to 37. Her glucose tolerance had improved, but her glucose levels were still a little on the high side. Despite her tremendous efforts, the lifestyle changes she had made hadn't eliminated all of her Syndrome X risk factors.

If the diet, exercise and lifestyle changes that you make are not enough to overcome Syndrome X, you may have to turn to medicine. But don't feel guilty or as if you've failed. Medicine is sometimes necessary, and if it's the right medicine, it may render Syndrome X harmless. Unfortunately, the wrong medicine can do you more harm than good. Let's take a look at the medicines you can use to combat Syndrome X, their pros and cons.

MEDICINE TO MAKE YOU MORE SENSITIVE TO YOUR INSULIN?

Syndrome X is triggered by a combination of insulin resistance and a resulting outpouring of insulin from the pancreas. Can the syndrome be defeated by making cells more sensitive to insulin?

Until relatively recently, doctors treated type 2 diabetes by giving patients either drugs that stimulated the pancreas to manufacture more insulin, or insulin itself. Attempting to stimulate pancreatic production of insulin is a rather crude approach. And while insulin injections work for most type 2 diabetics, they have side effects. Overdose, for example, can send blood sugar plummeting and bring on coma or death. More important, many patients just don't like all the bother that goes with daily injections.

A new approach was needed and, happily, it was found. In the last few years, the Food and Drug Administration (FDA) has approved a new class of drugs called "insulin sensitizers" to treat type 2 diabetes. By encouraging the diabetic's cells to respond to insulin's call to "open up" and take in the glucose, the medicine helps blood sugar fall to more normal levels. As an added plus, there is no need to worry about overdosing on insulin and falling into a coma, for insulin sensitizers simply make the insulin that's already present more effective; they don't add more.

The insulin sensitizers studied so far belong to a class of drugs called thiazolidenediones. Three of these have undergone large-scale clinical trials and demonstrated their ability to lower blood sugar levels in patients with type 2 diabetes, and the FDA has approved all three for clinical use. One of them, called trogltizone (trade name Rezulin), has been approved the longest, so we know more concerning its use in treating type 2 diabetes. Unfortunately, despite the many years devoted to evaluating its safety, the drug appears to have serious side effects involving the liver. The FDA has issued exhaustive guidelines mandating liver tests for patients being treated with Rezulin. The two other drugs, rosiglitazone (trade name Avanida) and pioglitazone (trade name Actos), have just recently received FDA approval. They appear to be less damaging to the liver, but they have not been used as long, or on as many people, as Rezulin. The best we can say is that they may well be safer, but only time will tell.

If the problem of liver damage caused by the thiazolidenediones were solved, it would seem that the next step is to use insulin sensitizers in the treatment of Syndrome X. After all, lack of insulin sensitivity is at the root of both type 2 diabetes and Syndrome X, so increasing sensitivity should solve both problems. And increasing insulin sensitivity would handle all the manifestations of Syndrome X with one fell swoop; you wouldn't need one drug for this manifestation and another for that.

Unfortunately, no one has yet conducted clinical trials to determine whether or not insulin sensitizers will help people with Syndrome X. These trials would have to show, first, that insulin sensitizers reduce insulin resistance and compensatory hyperinsulinemia, without unacceptable side effects, during the course of a six-to-twelve-month study. Then they would have to demonstrate that the drugs also lower the risk of heart attack in Syndrome X patients. (It's not enough to prove that they handle the insulin problems; the practical benefit, reducing the risk of heart disease, would also have to be shown.)

Conducting such complicated studies would require a tremendous investment from a major pharmaceutical company. But drug companies won't put up the money unless the world acknowledges that Syndrome X is a major cause of heart attacks—in other words, until there's a large, clear-cut market for these drugs. Until that happens, the idea of using insulin sensitizers for Syndrome X will have to remain an "orphan."

TREATING THE HYPERTRIGLYCERIDEMIA OF SYNDROME X

Although we don't have an "all-in-one" pill for Syndrome X, we can strike at its various manifestations. And since many of these are closely related, it is possible to treat several with one approach. For example, if the elevated blood fats (hypertriglyceridemia) seen with Syndrome X is reduced, other elements will improve greatly.

Triglyceride levels rarely rise unless one is suffering from both insulin resistance and compensatory hyperinsulinemia. Unfortunately, rising blood fats are a harbinger of terrible things to come. Once they start to climb, they will linger in the blood for longer periods of time (increased postprandial lipemia). You can also expect to see smaller and denser, hence more dangerous, LDL particles, plus lower levels of HDL "good" cholesterol.

If rising triglycerides are bad news, falling blood fats are just the opposite. When your triglyceride levels fall to normal levels, the fat in your blood will be cleared in a more timely manner following meals. What's more, you'll have greater amounts of HDL "good" cholesterol and be less likely to suffer from potentially fatal blood clots.

As you recall, people with Syndrome X have higher levels of PAI-1, which slows the dissolution of clots that can cause a heart attack. The higher your PAI-1, the more likely it is that an artery already damaged by Syndrome X will close off and trigger a heart attack. PAI-1 levels are higher in people with increased triglyceride concentrations, but they decrease when the triglyceride levels fall toward normal. This means that simply lowering blood fats reduces the risk of heart attack from high PAI-1 levels.

The FDA has approved three drugs to lower triglyceride levels. One of them, nicotinic acid, has been available for years and works quite well, slowing the release of fatty acids from fat cells. (The liver uses fatty acids to manufacture triglyceride-rich VLDL, so with fewer fatty acids at its disposal, the liver makes less VLDL and blood fat levels drop.) Nicotinic acid also lowers LDL cholesterol.

Surprisingly, despite nicotinic acid's double benefits, doctors rarely prescribe it. This is primarily because within 15 to 20 minutes of taking nicotinic acid, many patients suffer an unpleasant flushing sensation to the face that feels much like a sunburn and can last for up to an hour. Patients also occasionally complain of feeling lightheaded. These side effects are triggered by nicotinic acid's ability to dilate blood vessels all over the body, particularly in the skin. These problems can often be handled by starting with small amounts of the medicine and slowly increasing the dosage as the symptoms go away. Nevertheless, some patients are unable to tolerate the drug, no matter how valiantly they try.

In addition to nicotinic acid, two other medicines, both members of the fibric acid class of drugs, lower blood fats. They are gemfibrozil (trade name Lopid) and fenofibrate (Tricor). These drugs have been used extensively in Europe. Gemfibrozil has been available in the United States for years, and the FDA has recently approved fenofibrate. Both drugs lower blood fats by decreasing the liver's production of VLDL, and by increasing the rate at which triglyceride-rich lipoproteins are removed from the blood. Although people usually tolerate both of these drugs very well, it's a good idea to have your liver function tested at regular intervals, just to be safe.

KEEPING YOUR BLOOD PRESSURE IN CHECK

We have known for many years that patients with high blood pressure are at a greatly increased risk of heart attack, stroke or both, whether or not they have Syndrome X. Not surprisingly, several large-scale clinical trials have shown that lowering blood pressure will significantly decrease the risk from both. What is surprising, though, is that the drugs used to lower blood pressure are better at reducing the risk of stroke than heart attack. We don't really know why this is, although we do know that 50 percent of patients with high blood pressure are also insulin resistant, with increased insulin levels in their blood and many other manifestations of Syndrome X. Moreover, it seems to be precisely these patients who are at the greatest risk of heart attack! Obviously, there is a connection between hypertension and Syndrome X, and a great need for those with Syndrome X to get their blood pressure under control.

The last decade has seen a dramatic increase in the number of drugs that treat hypertension. In fact, today there are so many effective drugs for hypertension that there is absolutely no reason for anyone's blood pressure to remain uncontrolled.

There are five different chemical classes of drugs used to treat hypertension, all of which have been approved by the FDA: diuretics, beta blockers, alpha blockers, calcium channel blockers and ACE inhibitors. Within each of these five classes there are multiple FDA-approved drugs, all about equally effective. These drugs are far too numerous to discuss each one individually, but we can briefly explain how each class works, and mention some common side effects.

Diuretics

Long known for safely and effectively lowering blood pressure, diuretics are believed to work primarily by helping to reduce the amount of salt and water in the body. This reduces the blood volume, which means there's less blood flowing through the pipes and thus lower pressure.

Diuretics are effective but have disadvantages, including the loss of potassium and increasing risk of type 2 diabetes in individuals at risk. Moreover, they can increase triglyceride and lower HDL cholesterol levels, which is exactly what you don't want, especially if you have Syndrome X. Diuretics can also impair sexual function in males.

If you are taking a diuretic, have your blood tested for plasma potassium, glucose and lipid levels at regular intervals. The higher the dose of a diuretic, the greater the risk of side effects, so smaller doses are better, consistent with good health. The dose required to lower blood pressure is much lower than that which can bring on side effects.

Beta Blockers

These drugs also have a long, successful track record in treating hypertension. Beta blockers act by binding to specific receptors on the nerve endings that control the width (caliber) of your blood vessels, and by slowing the heart rate.

Widening the blood vessels makes it easier for blood to flow, while slowing of the heart rate reduces the amount of "push" driving the blood through the arteries and veins. Together, these two actions reduce the blood pressure. Moreover, beta blockers will decrease the level of hormones called catecholamines, which cause blood vessels to constrict (narrow).

Beta blockers are particularly effective in those who have had heart attacks; studies show that their use prolongs life after heart attack. However, the beta blockers have side effects, the most common of which is fatigue. The drugs can also increase plasma glucose and lipid levels, and impair sexual function in men.

Alpha Blockers

Like the beta blockers, alpha blockers lower blood pressure by binding to specific receptors on nerve endings. In doing so, they interfere with the normal flow of signals that make arteries constrict. The arteries widen (dilate) and the blood flows more freely.

Unlike the diuretics and beta blockers, alpha blockers don't adversely affect glucose, lipids or sexual function, and they may actually improve insulin sensitivity. However, these essentially side-effect-free drugs that could be so beneficial for people with Syndrome X are infrequently prescribed for hypertension. Physicians don't seem nearly as aware of the benefits of these drugs as they should be, probably because the first FDA-approved alpha blocker was short-acting and could cause blood pressure to fall too drastically. The problem has disappeared with the appearance of approved long-acting alpha blockers, and their use is slowly increasing.

Calcium Channel Blockers

Physicians initially prescribed calcium channel blockers to treat angina pectoris (chest pain associated with coronary artery disease). Today, they are commonly used for hypertension. Calcium channel blockers block the entry of calcium (which blood vessel cells need in order to constrict) into the cells. The blood vessels then dilate, offering less resistance to the flow of blood, and blood pressure falls.

There are many different drugs in this class, all of which are able to lower blood pressure without increasing any of the manifestations of Syndrome X. They do, however, have side effects, which vary from drug to drug. Some of the common side effects are headaches, flushing and swelling of the ankles.

Angiotensin-Converting Enzyme (ACE) Inhibitors

Angiotensin is a powerful hormone that increases blood pressure by constricting the arteries. In order for the body to make this hormone, its inactive precursor must be "converted" to angiotensin by angiotensin-converting enzyme (ACE).

ACE inhibitors decrease the ability of ACE to produce angiotensin, thus preventing the body from making as much of this hormone as it otherwise would. With less angiotensin in circulation, arteries and blood vessels constrict less, blood flow improves and blood pressure falls. The FDA has approved many effective ACE inhibitors, which have also been shown to be very helpful in treating heart failure.

ACE inhibitors lower blood pressure with few, if any, side effects, and they will not make Syndrome X worse. The most common side effect is a chronic dry cough, which occurs in about 15 percent of all patients taking the drug. The problem is not serious, but can be annoying enough to cause a patient to stop taking the medication. Unfortunately, switching to a different ACE inhibitor will not resolve the problem.

As of this writing, there are new drugs that seek to influence angiotensin in a different way. Instead of interfering with the production of the hormone, they block angiotensin receptors on certain cells, preventing the hormone from constricting arteries and raising blood pressure. But whether or not these new drugs will be more useful than ACE inhibitors in the treatment of hypertension remains to be seen.

GO ALL THE WAY AND CAST A WIDE NET

Keep two important principles in mind when treating high blood pressure as part of Syndrome X. First, get that pressure low enough to make a real difference. Once you begin treatment, stay with it until your pressure is below 140/90. Second, remember that you'll need to address all of the Syndrome X factors, not just hypertension.

In many cases, a single anti-hypertensive drug won't do the trick; a combination of two or three drugs may be required. Fortunately, drugs from all five classes (diuretics, alpha blockers, beta blockers, calcium channel blockers and ACE inhibitors) can be combined, and it is highly likely that the right "formula" can be found for you.

Of course, drugs that lower blood pressure only work if you take them regularly. When medicines fail, it's not usually because the patient's hypertension is too "tough." More commonly, it's because he or she isn't taking the medicine regularly.

When you find the right medication or combination of medications that keeps your blood pressure in check, remember that you must simultaneously attack *all* the risk factors for Syndrome X. Get tested for the other abnormalities seen with the syndrome and begin preparing your health plan. Test results should show:

- your blood sugar level after an overnight fast
- your blood sugar level two hours after a 75 gram oral glucose challenge
- your fasting level of blood fats (plasma triglycerides)
- your LDL "bad" cholesterol level
- your HDL "good" cholesterol level

If all of these values are well within normal range, you may do well with any one of the anti-hypertensive drugs, as all are approximately equal in terms of blood-pressure-lowering ability.

If, however, your values are abnormal, you and your doctor must select your blood pressure medication more carefully. The more abnormal your blood tests are, the more important it will be to find just the right drug or combination of drugs. For example, diuretics and beta blockers can worsen both glucose tolerance and blood lipid levels, so it's probably best to avoid these kinds of drugs if your laboratory results are anything less than perfectly normal. (But if you have had a heart attack, the benefits of beta blockers may outweigh their potentially harmful metabolic effects.)

The three remaining classes of anti-hypertensive drugs (alpha blockers, calcium channel blockers and ACE inhibitors) are much less likely to accentuate the abnormalities of Syndrome X, so any of these may be right for you. The main consideration may be your triglyceride levels. The higher your triglycerides, the more beneficial it may be to begin treatment with an alpha blocker, which won't adversely affect your lipid levels.

If your blood pressure does not fall below 140/90 in response to one anti-hypertensive drug, talk to your doctor about adding a second. Generally speaking, the guidelines listed above for selecting the first blood pressure medicine will also apply to the second. However, if you began with an ACE inhibitor, adding a *low* dose of a diuretic can have an extremely beneficial effect on blood pressure. And because no one needs to take more than a low dose of a diuretic to lower blood pressure, there are no harmful metabolic effects to worry about.

Some pills contain both an ACE inhibitor and a *low*-dose diuretic. Unfortunately, it is not possible to obtain a pill that contains *just* a low dose of a diuretic in the United States. If we could get such a drug, it would be useful as a first and single drug in patients with abnormal glucose and/or lipid metabolism. But since the low-dose diuretic is not available as a single medication, avoid diuretics as the first choice of medicine if you have any of the metabolic abnormalities mentioned above.

DON'T IGNORE A HIGH LDL CHOLESTEROL

Although a high LDL "bad" cholesterol level is not part of Syndrome X, it shouldn't be ignored. Elevated LDL is an important risk factor for heart attack all by itself, and the danger increases when you have a high LDL cholesterol plus Syndrome X. Read through the dietary information in Chapter 6 to see how you can keep your LDL "bad" cholesterol as low as your genetic legacy permits.

If your LDL cholesterol remains above 130 mg/dl despite dietary changes, the American Heart Association recommends that you take medication to lower it. If you have a high LDL *and* other risk factors for heart attack, you should get it down below 130. For example, if you have a high LDL combined with high blood pressure, you should try to get your LDL down to less than 100 mg/dl.

Fortunately, drugs are available now that can help lower LDL cholesterol. All of these drugs inhibit an enzyme involved in cellular cholesterol metabolism, and they all lead to an increase in the liver's ability to remove cholesterol from the blood. As a result, your LDL cholesterol concentration will fall. Studies have shown that these drugs are highly effective in reducing heart attacks.

IN SHORT

Drugs can and do work wonders. Nevertheless, it's preferable to begin by making lifestyle changes, which by themselves are often enough to reduce the risk of heart attack. If you've tried your best with lifestyle changes but the results are not good enough, medications are appropriate. Fortunately, we now have very effective drugs available that can help prevent coronary heart disease. Relying on medication to lower your risk of heart attack doesn't mean you've failed. If you've adopted the healthiest lifestyle possible and it still isn't enough, complementing your lifestyle changes with the careful and prudent use of drugs to reduce the odds of suffering a heart attack makes perfect sense.

BEYOND SYNDROME X

SO FAR, WE'VE FOCUSED ON using the six-step program to overcome Syndrome X and lessen your risk of heart attack. But the program does more; its beneficial "side effects" include reducing your risk of developing obesity, type 2 diabetes and hypercholesterolemia, conditions that can trigger a heart attack and other problems. And as you combat obesity you'll enjoy even more "side effects," including reducing your risk of joint problems, lowering high blood pressure and avoiding gallbladder disease. So even if you don't have Syndrome X, the six-step program can be beneficial.

THE SIX-STEP PROGRAM FIGHTS OBESITY

The incidence of obesity in developed countries has reached epidemic proportions. To put it bluntly, as a nation we're fat. Alarmed by our growing girth, the United States government conducted a series of health surveys to track our sorry "progress." From the 1962 National Health Examination Survey (NHES) through 1994's National Health and Nutrition Examination Survey III (NHANES III), we've gotten fatter and fatter. The chart on page 144 shows the rise in the percentage of Americans who are either obese or overweight, according to four key surveys. In the early 1960s, 13 percent of us were obese and 43 percent overweight. By the mid-1990s, the figures had jumped to 22 percent obese and 54 percent overweight.

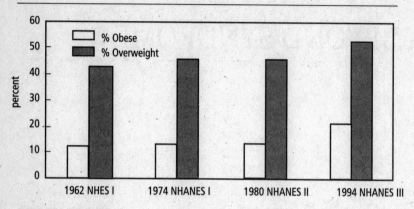

A Growing Problem

The 1962 National Health Examination Survey (NHES I) and three National Health and Nutrition Examination Surveys (NHANES I, II and III) have tracked the growing problems of overweight and obesity in this country.

If we consider only those people who are overweight,[1] not obese, here's how some of the numbers break down:

- 104.4 million American adults are overweight.
- Among non-Hispanic white adults (ages 20 to 74), 59.6 percent of men and 45.5 percent of women are overweight.
- Among non-Hispanic black adults, 57.5 percent of men and 66.5 percent of women are overweight.
- Among Mexican-American adults, 67.1 percent of men and 67.6 percent of women are overweight.

How about obesity? Here are some statistics for this more dangerous condition:[2]

- 42.5 million American adults are obese.
- Among non-Hispanic white adults, 20 percent of men and 22.4 percent of women are obese.

[1] Those who have a body mass index (BMI) of 25 to 30.
[2] Obesity is defined in these studies as BMIs of 30 or more.

- Among non-Hispanic black adults, 21.3 percent of men and 37.4 percent of women are obese.
- Among Mexican-American adults, 23.1 percent of men and 34.2 percent of women are obese.

The danger of obesity is built right into its definition. According to the 1985 National Institutes of Health Consensus Development Conference, obesity "is an excess of body fat frequently resulting in a significant impairment in health."

Figuring the Fat with Body Mass Index (BMI)

How many extra pounds can you carry without being considered obese? For many years we relied on life insurance tables to determine whether or not someone was obese. These tables, which simply gave acceptable weight ranges for each sex according to height and frame size, were a good start. Unfortunately, they were subjective and somewhat vague. For example, it wasn't clear how to determine whether you had a small, medium or large frame. Looking for a more objective method of defining obesity, the scientific community came up with the body mass index (BMI).

To calculate your BMI, divide your body weight (in kilograms) by your height (in meters) squared. This formula sounds difficult for those of us used to thinking in terms of pounds, feet and inches, rather than kilograms and meters, but it's fairly simple once you lay out the steps. Suppose a man is 5 feet 10 inches tall and weighs 220 pounds:

1. Convert weight into kilograms. One kilogram equals 2.2 pounds, so divide 220 pounds by 2.2, to get 100 kilograms.
2. Convert height to inches. Five feet 10 inches equals 70 inches.
3. Then convert height in inches to meters. One meter equals 39.37 inches. If you have a calculator, go ahead and divide the height in inches by 39.37. Otherwise, round 39.37 off to 40 and divide: 70 inches divided by 40 equals 1.75 meters.
4. Square the height in meters by multiplying it by itself. 1.75 times 1.75 equals 3.06 meters.
5. Divide the weight in kilograms (step 1) by the height in meters squared (step 4): 100 divided by 3.06 equals 32.6

There you have it. The 5-foot 10-inch man has a BMI of 32.6, and would be considered obese.

Here's another example, a woman weighing 130 pounds and standing 5 feet 4 inches.

1. Convert weight into kilograms. One kilogram equals 2.2 pounds, so 130 pounds divided by 2.2 equals 59.1 kilograms.
2. Convert height to inches. Five feet 4 inches equals 64 inches.
3. Convert height in inches to meters: 64 inches divided by 40 equals 1.6 meters.
4. Square the height in meters by multiplying it by itself: 1.6 times 1.6 equals 2.56 meters.
5. Divide the weight in kilograms (step 1) by the height in meters squared (step 4): 59.1 divided by 2.56 equals 23.1.

Standing 6 inches shorter and 90 pounds lighter than the man in the previous example, this woman has a BMI of 23.1. She is neither overweight nor obese.

Calculate Your BMI

Your weight in pounds is _____
Your height in feet and inches is _____

1. Convert weight to kilograms.
(Divide your weight in pounds by 2.2.)
_____ ÷ 2.2 = _____ kilograms

2. Convert your height to inches.
Height in feet multiplied by 12 inches = _____ + any remaining inches = _____ total inches height

3. Convert height in inches to meters.
(Divide the result of step 2 by 40.)
Total inches in height _____ ÷ 40 = _____ total meters in height

4. Square the height in meters by multiplying it by itself.
(Multiply the result of step 3 by itself.)
Total meters in height _____ x total meters in height _____ = _____ meters

5. Divide the weight in kilograms by the height in meters squared.
(Divide the result of step 1 by the result of step 4.)
_____ kilograms of weight ÷ _____ meters = _____ = BMI

What Should the BMI Be?

Interpreting the BMI is quite simple. Some authorities feel that men should be considered obese when their BMIs are 30 or greater, and women when their numbers rise above 28.6. I'm stricter because excess pounds can be especially dangerous to those with Syndrome X. Here are the guidelines I favor, and the steps you should take in each range. (These ranges are designed for both men and women.)

- You're in the SAFETY range with a BMI of 25 or less. Congratulations! You do not need to lose weight. Focus on healthful eating and exercise rather than on counting calories.
- You're in the CAUTION range with a BMI of 26. You're flirting with danger. Watch your intake and slice off a few calories every day, starting now.
- You're in the CONCERN range with a BMI of 27 to 29. This is not good news. You're overweight and need to get serious about slimming down. Begin shedding those excess pounds now with exercise and the Syndrome X Diet.
- You're in the DANGER range with a BMI of 30 or greater. You're significantly overweight and your risk of heart attack is substantially increased. Tell your doctor about your plans to begin your exercise program. Discuss your physical condition and any medical problems, as well your plans to go on the Syndrome X Diet.

The Difference Is Slight

Composition studies have shown that women's bodies naturally have more fat than men's. Consequently, at any given BMI, women will be somewhat more "fatty" than men. However, the differences between men and women are so slight that the BMI ranges work equally well for both sexes.

Although the BMI is an improvement over the simple height-weight charts, it's not perfect. A football player, boxer or weight lifter may have a "high" BMI because he's well muscled and muscles weigh a lot. An athlete and a couch potato of similar size and weight may have similar BMIs, but very different amounts of body fat. The BMI is an excellent gauge for most of us, but body composition studies may be necessary to fine-tune the assessment for some people.

The Health Costs of Obesity

According to the 1994 NHANES III figures, a whopping 50 percent of Americans are overweight, some 22 percent of those between the ages of twenty and seventy-four are obese, and the incidence of obesity in the United States doubled between 1962 and 1994. How does all of this extra poundage harm our health? It certainly increases the risk of Syndrome X, but that's not all. Obesity is a contributing factor to coronary heart disease, joint problems, type 2 diabetes, hypertension, gall bladder disease and menstrual disorders. And that's just the short list.

The American Heart Association reported on a study[3] that compared the level of obesity to the risk of developing heart disease in men and women. The results were not surprising—greater pounds equal greater risk. For men the odds of suffering heart disease were:

- Not obese (BMI of 22.5)—35 percent chance
- Mildly obese (BMI of 27.5)—38 percent
- Moderately obese (BMI of 32.5)—42 percent
- Severely obese (BMI of 37.5)—46 percent

For women the odds were:

- Not obese—25 percent chance
- Mildly obese—29 percent
- Moderately obese—32 percent
- Severely obese—37 percent

The researchers went beyond damage to the heart to see how obesity hurts the wallet. Notice how the average expected medical costs for treatment of heart disease rose in lockstep with increasing obesity. For men:

- Not obese—$10,500 average expected lifetime cost
- Mildly obese—$12,000

[3] "Lifetime risks and costs of heart disease much higher for obese." American Heart Association Abstract #2519, November 10, 1998.

- Moderately obese—$14,000
- Severely obese—$16,400

For women the costs were:

- Not obese—$5,800
- Mildly obese—$6,700
- Moderately obese—$7,900
- Severely obese—$9,400

Here are some of the other serious side effects of obesity that most concern the National Institutes of Health:[4]

- *Hypertension.* Being overweight makes you almost three times more likely to develop elevated blood pressure. And the risk is even higher for overweight adults between the ages of twenty and forty-four, who are more than five times as likely to suffer the effects of this "silent killer" as their thinner counterparts. Numerous studies have shown a direct link between pounds and pressure: blood pressure goes up as the pounds pile on, and drops as the weight is shed.
- *Diabetes.* This devastating crippler and killer is almost three times as likely to strike the overweight as it is those of normal weight.
- *Psychological distress.* Many overweight and obese people suffer psychologically, feeling depressed, worthless and out of control. They may become uncomfortable, embarrassed and socially withdrawn.
- *Early death.* Several studies, including the American Cancer Society Study and the Framingham Thirty-Year Follow-up Study, have found that obesity can cut life short. The more obese one is, the greater the risk of early death.

Even if you don't have Syndrome X, being either overweight or obese is both dangerous and expensive. Use the six-step program to slim down the healthy way.

[4] "Implications of Obesity." NIH Consensus Statement 1985 February 11–13; 5(9):1–7. See also AHA Conference Proceeding. "Obesity: Impact on Cardiovascular Disease." R. M. Krauss, M. Winston, B. J. Fletcher, conference codirectors. Reprint No. 71-0152.

Fat Facts

- Between the ages of twenty-five and fifty-five, the average American puts on twenty pounds.
- Adults take in some 900,000 to 1,000,000 calories per year.
- According to the American Heart Association,* women with a higher level of education are slimmer on average than lesser-educated women, but education level seems to have no effect on men's girth.
- We spend an awful lot of money trying to slim down: well over $30 billion per year on medically supervised weight loss programs, diet sodas, gyms and health clubs, diet dinners and other meals, treadmills and other exercise equipment.†

* AHA Conference Proceeding, "Obesity: Impact on Cardiovascular Disease," R. M. Krauss, M. Winston, B. J. Fletcher, conference codirectors. Reprint No. 71-0152.

† Ibid.

THE SIX-STEP PROGRAM GUARDS AGAINST TYPE 2 DIABETES AND "PRE-DIABETES"

Approximately 16 million Americans have type 2 diabetes, although almost half of them don't realize it. At least twice as many people have impaired glucose tolerance (IGT)—"pre-diabetes"—and don't know it.

Both type 2 diabetes and IGT are serious problems. When you have IGT, your blood sugar (plasma glucose) levels are higher than normal. Not high enough to qualify you as being diabetic, but you're in dangerous territory. Each year, about 5 percent of those with IGT "graduate" to type 2 diabetes. But even if you don't "graduate," you're not safe, for the vast majority of those with IGT will have manifestations of Syndrome X.

The number of Americans with type 2 diabetes or IGT is growing at an alarming rate. We need to get these potentially crippling diseases under control, and can do so by adopting the Six-Step Syndrome X Program.

Why Are We Suffering More?

It's safe to say that modern Western living and type 2 diabetes go hand in hand. In fact, the more economically developed a nation, the more likely its people are to have this problem. This is because improved medical treatment and a higher standard of living allow us to live longer, while labor-saving devices afford us more leisure time and diminish the need to engage in physical activity. Our lives have become increasingly sedentary: most of us work in offices or shops, rather than on farms or in factories. Most of us ride to work, rather than walk. Most of us warm our homes by turning up the heater, rather than chopping wood or shoveling coal. Most of us don't even have to get up from our easy chairs to change the channel on the television; we simply push a button on the remote control. But this lack of activity combined with our propensity toward living longer lives has proven to be a major cause of both type 2 diabetes and Syndrome X. Here's why:

- The pancreas's ability to secrete insulin likely declines with age, and we are living longer than ever.
- Physical inactivity sets the stage for obesity, and most of us tend to become even more sedentary as we age.
- The obese are more likely to develop type 2 diabetes, and on average we are heavier today than we have ever been.
- The more sedentary and the heavier we are, the more insulin resistance we develop.

More difficulty secreting insulin, less physical activity, a higher incidence of obesity and more insulin resistance all add up to a much greater risk of type 2 diabetes.

A Quiet Crippler and Killer

The seventh leading cause of death in the United States, type 2 diabetes is most often "silent." That's one of the worst things about the disease—you may not know anything is amiss until you go in for a routine checkup, or you're in the hospital because of a car accident, a ruptured appendix or perhaps a heart attack.

Whether it creeps in silently or announces its presence, diabetes can cause a great deal of trouble. Just as the excess insulin in the bloodstream seen with Syndrome X causes wide-ranging damage, the large amounts of blood sugar characteristic of diabetes affect tissues and organs all over the body. Complications of the disease include:

- *Heart disease.* Diabetes encourages the buildup of plaque in the coronary arteries, which can lead to a heart attack. Having diabetes increases the risk of heart disease two to four times.
- *Kidney damage.* Chronic increases in blood sugar concentrations lead to poor kidney function and eventual kidney failure. Diabetes is the primary cause of end-stage renal disease and dialysis.
- *Blindness.* Vision suffers as the blood vessels in the retina are damaged. Diabetes is the primary cause of blindness among people aged twenty to seventy-four.
- *Stroke.* Damage to the arteries in the brain increases the diabetic's risk of stroke two to four times.
- *Nerve damage.* If the nerves are affected, there may be weakness, tingling or a numbing sensation in the parts of the body served by the damaged nerve(s). Numbness, which commonly strikes diabetics in the feet, can be especially dangerous because people may not be aware that they've hurt themselves. Improperly fitting shoes or careless trimming of the toenails may cause injury to the feet that they don't even notice. To make matters worse, the poor circulation commonly seen with diabetes causes poor wound healing and may allow infection to set in, which can lead to gangrene and possible amputation. Diabetics have a greatly increased risk of losing a foot or leg to amputation.
- *Gastrointestinal disorders.* If the nerves controlling digestion are injured, diabetics may have difficulty swallowing, digesting food and/or absorbing nutrients. Chronic diarrhea and other gastrointestinal difficulties can ensue.
- *Sexual problems.* Due to nerve damage and poor circulation, diabetic men frequently suffer from erectile dysfunction.

Clearly, diabetes is a serious problem. The Syndrome X program won't directly help type 1 diabetics, for they must take insulin for the rest of their lives. However, the six-step program can be a boon for those with type 2—which is the vast majority of diabetics. Rigorously following the program will help prevent this form of diabetes. And for those who have it, the program can improve or even eliminate all of the manifestations of the disease.

If you have type 2 diabetes, you won't have to change the Six-Step Syndrome X Program in any way. Just follow the guidelines and you'll help control both diabetes and impaired glucose tolerance.

Diabetes Dollars and Cents

As the number of patients with type 2 diabetes rises, the human and economic costs mount. If you're middle-aged, having type 2 diabetes can shorten your life expectancy by five to ten years, quite likely through a heart attack.

Diabetes takes a serious toll in the workplace. Workers aged eighteen to sixty-four with diabetes lost an average of 8.3 days from work in 1997. That compares to only 1.7 work days lost by people who did not have the disease. In the same year, almost 75,000 workers were permanently disabled by diabetes.

What's the price tag for diabetes and its side effects? The dollar cost of treatment and loss of productivity related to type 2 diabetes is estimated to have been *$98 billion* in 1997.* And it's only going up.

* "Diabetes Info: Diabetes Facts and Figures," American Diabetes Association, 1997, www.diabetes.org/default.asp.

THE SIX-STEP PROGRAM VERSUS HYPERCHOLESTEROLEMIA

Hypercholesterolemia is a big word describing elevated concentrations of the "bad" LDL cholesterol in the bloodstream. Excess LDL is a major risk factor for heart attack, unrelated to Syndrome X.

It may be confusing at first to hear that elevated LDL cholesterol is separate from Syndrome X because one of the risk factors of Syndrome X is smaller and denser LDL particles. Syndrome X does, in fact, affect the nature of your LDL particles, but not how much LDL cholesterol is in your system in the first place.

If you have elevated LDL cholesterol but none of the other manifestations of Syndrome X, you are almost certainly insulin-sensitive and don't have to worry that leftover high insulin levels are ravaging your body. However, it is not uncommon for a person to have a double whammy: *both* elevated LDL cholesterol and one or more elements of Syndrome X. People with both conditions have the highest risk of heart attack.

What Makes LDL Rise?

Differing genetic makeup probably accounts for about 80 percent of the difference in LDL levels from person to person, with variations in lifestyle contributing only 20 percent. This doesn't mean that we can't lower our LDL cholesterol, but our genes limit what we can do through lifestyle changes. Fortunately, we have powerful medicines that can help lower LDL cholesterol if changes in diet and exercise aren't enough.

If insulin resistance doesn't push up LDL cholesterol, what does? The problem seems to lie in the number of LDL receptors on the surface of most, if not all, of the body's cells. These receptors help your body clear LDL from the bloodstream. If your "genetic instruction sheet" includes too few receptors, or inefficient ones, you will have difficulty removing LDL cholesterol from your blood, and your levels will rise. However, no matter how many LDL receptors you have and how efficient they are, eating more saturated fat will slow the removal process.

What do you eat instead? If you have Syndrome X, replace saturated fats with unsaturated ones. If you're only suffering from elevated LDL, you can replace saturated fats with unsaturated fats and/or carbohydrate.

The Syndrome X Diet makes the issue simple for you. It is nutritious and health-enhancing for everyone—for those who have Syndrome X, those who have elevated LDL cholesterol, and those who have both or neither. It lowers LDL cholesterol and reduces the manifestations of Syndrome X.

One Program with Many Benefits

The six-step program is the only complete way to protect yourself from Syndrome X. And whether or not you have the syndrome, you can use the program to fight obesity, type 2 diabetes and hypercholesterolemia, as well as the joint problems, hypertension, gallbladder disease, menstrual disorders and other ailments associated with too much weight. The six-step program is just about everyone's ticket to better health.

IF YOU HAVE

HEART DISEASE

THIS YEAR, HUNDREDS OF thousands of Americans will rush to their doctor's offices or to emergency rooms suffering from the chest pain and/or other problems associated with coronary heart disease. Over one million Americans will actually suffer a heart attack, and more than a third of them will die. The ones who make it through the harrowing experience, however, are not yet "home free." Even those who survive a heart attack may be struck by "side effects" such as congestive heart failure, persistent irregular heartbeat, stroke and blood clots in the heart, legs or elsewhere.

The graph on the next page shows the sobering heart disease death statistics for 1995.

I wrote this book to introduce you to an important, poorly recognized cause of heart attack, and to provide you with the information needed to maximally decrease your chance of suffering such an attack. Unfortunately, no program is 100 percent successful. Despite your best efforts, you may develop a degree of coronary heart disease that makes a heart attack more likely. In this chapter I will describe the kinds of tests your doctor may do to gauge your degree of heart disease, as well as treatments currently being used to prevent active heart attacks in those who are on the brink of developing them.

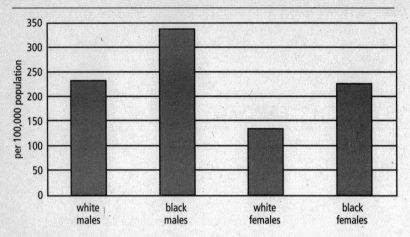

Age-Adjusted Coronary Heart Disease Death Rates in the U.S., 1995

Although the death rates from coronary heart disease are too high for everyone, black males are especially at risk.

Some people think they have plenty of time before they need worry about heart disease, that their bodies will give ample warning. After all, they've heard countless stories of people clutching at their chests in pain, yet living to tell about it, and since they're not hurting now, they feel they must be OK. Unfortunately, heart disease is often "silent." Approximately one-third of all attacks strike without pain or other warning. The first sign of trouble may be the heart attack itself.

Whether induced by Syndrome X or not, heart disease is a serious problem requiring immediate care. It doesn't hurt to have your heart checked out by a physician before trouble strikes, especially if you are already experiencing the chest pain that may be telling you that trouble is on its way. Typically, the kind of chest pain that warns of a heart attack is felt under your breastbone, or to the left of that area. It is often precipitated by exertion, or may strike after you eat a large meal. The sensation can be quite painful, but is often described as a feeling of great pressure. The pain may stay in the same place, or might radiate to your left arm or jaw. It typically lasts for only a few minutes, and goes away as you stop the activity that precipitated it.

The pain is due to a decrease in the flow of blood from the coronary arteries, and the resulting lack of oxygen delivered to your heart muscle. It often occurs with exercise because blood is diverted from the heart to the muscles, or after a large meal, when blood is shunted to the intestinal track. In either case, the great need for blood elsewhere strains the body's ability to get enough blood to the coronary arteries feeding the heart.

If you feel any suspicious chest pain, visit your physician to make sure of the cause. And even if you don't have chest pain, it makes sense to schedule an appointment with your physician to evaluate your heart if you:

- have any of the manifestations of Syndrome X
- are a male age forty-five or older
- are a postmenopausal female
- are overweight or obese
- have a family history of heart disease, high blood pressure or diabetes
- have a total serum cholesterol over 200 mg/dl, particularly if it's over 240 mg/dl and coupled with an LDL cholesterol over 130 mg/dl
- have an HDL cholesterol less than 35 mg/dl and a triglyceride greater than 200 mg/dl
- smoke

LOOKING AT THE HEART

The symptoms of a heart attack—crushing chest pain, difficulty breathing, nausea, sweating and more—are alarming. But the diagnosis of heart attack isn't always obvious, because it's not the only thing that can cause these problems. Heartburn, for example, can trigger severe pain in the chest and neck. On the other hand, actual heart attacks may produce no symptoms, or only very mild ones that are mistaken for heartburn, fatigue or an upset stomach.

Rather than send everyone with symptoms into surgery for a bypass operation, doctors must carefully evaluate patients to see whose heart is really under siege, and what care is appropriate. Unless you are in the throes of a heart attack or another problem, your doctor should perform a careful and thorough examination, verifying that you do indeed have coronary heart disease.

A variety of tests can be used to provide information about the heart, including the electrocardiogram (EKG), echocardiogram, exercise stress test and cardiac catheterization. Let's take a brief look at each.

Electrocardiogram (EKG)

This is one of the simplest ways for doctors to "see" how the heart behaves. A little bit of gel is used to stick several electrodes to your chest and limbs while you lie on a table. The electrodes monitor the electrical activity of your heart, providing information about the way your heart beats and the way the heart muscle functions, indicating whether or not you've had a heart attack. There are no side effects to EKGs, which can be performed right in your doctor's office.

Echocardiogram

If the physical examination and electrocardiogram do not provide your doctor with the information needed to make a definitive diagnosis, he or she may call for an echocardiogram. This harmless procedure, very similar to the ultrasound routinely performed on pregnant women, gives the doctor an "inside" look at your heart.

The procedure is very simple. A technician will hook you up to an electrocardiograph, then smear an odorless gel on your chest. Next, he or she will hold a transducer (a device that looks something like a microphone) up to the skin above or near your heart. This transducer will generate and "broadcast" sound waves into your heart, receive the sound waves that bounce back, then translate them into pictures of your heart. You'll be asked to lie still during this test, which takes forty-five minutes to an hour, and occasionally to hold your breath, inhaling or exhaling upon request. The procedure is painless and harmless, and you may be able to watch images of your heart on a television screen.

By studying the images on the screen (as well as those recorded on paper and videotape), your doctor can gauge how well your heart pumps blood, how the valves between your heart chambers work, how your blood flows through your heart, how large your heart chambers are, whether or not there are any blood clots in the chambers and what the insides of the arteries look like.

Stress Test

Also known as a stress electrocardiogram and exercise tolerance test, this procedure takes the EKG a step further. The EKG shows how your heart functions while you're lying down in the doctor's office. But how does it perform when you're putting extra demands on your heart by moving actively? The only way to tell is to get moving and see.

Your physician may call for this test to see if you have coronary heart disease or other heart problems. If you do have coronary heart disease, this test can help your doctor determine the severity. Your doctor may also request an exercise stress test following coronary artery bypass surgery or balloon angioplasty to help devise an effective—and safe—rehabilitation program.

The test itself is fairly simple, though strenuous. Electrodes will be placed on your body, and a blood pressure cuff will be attached to your arm. A resting EKG and blood pressure will be taken, then you'll be asked to walk on a treadmill. You'll start slowly, with the doctor increasing the speed as well as the pitch of the treadmill, tilting it so you'll be walking uphill as the test progresses.

Throughout the exercise tolerance test, the doctor will monitor your blood pressure and electrocardiogram, looking for signs that your heart is not receiving enough oxygen.

It's perfectly normal to feel tired or short of breath or to sweat during the test. After all, you will be walking (possibly quite rapidly) on a treadmill that may be tilted up. However, chest pain or unusual shortness of breath are danger signs. Be sure to tell your physician if you feel faint, dizzy or unusually fatigued, if there is pain or discomfort in your chest, jaw or arm, if you are having difficulty breathing or if your leg muscles are sore or cramped.

When you've finished exercising, the doctor will leave the electrodes and blood pressure cuff in place for another ten minutes or so to continue the monitoring.

Preparation for the test is simple. Your doctor will instruct you not to eat, drink or smoke for several hours before the test, and will talk to you about any medications you are currently taking. You'll be asked to wear comfortable clothing and sneakers or other rubber-soled shoes. Since you may have to undress from the waist up, women may be advised to wear a two-piece outfit.

The test is noninvasive; that is, no cuts are made in your skin, and nothing is put into your body or taken out. Neither are there any drug side effects to worry about. However, the exercise may trigger problems if you have coronary heart disease or certain other conditions. You may become dizzy, feel pain or become short of breath during the test. It's possible that you might even suffer a heart attack during the test, although the odds of that happening are slight. Your doctor will want to know about any conditions that may make the test too dangerous to take, including certain abnormal heart rhythms, severe congestive heart failure or elevated blood pressure, heart infections or valve disease, or any other condition that prevents you from exercising safely.

The *stress echocardiogram* is very similar to the exercise stress test, with the addition of an echocardiogram to allow the physician an extra look at your heart. You'll be hooked up to electrodes and asked to exercise on the treadmill. Then, when your heart is beating at a certain level, you'll lie down for the echocardiogram.

The *nuclear stress test* is another variation of the exercise stress test, the difference being that toward the end of the test, you'll be given a small injection of thallium or another radioactive material. Then, while you're lying down, a gamma-ray camera will be passed over your body, taking pictures of your thallium-lit heart in action, still "revved up" from exercising on the treadmill.

Several hours later, you'll be given another injection of thallium and the gamma-ray camera will take pictures of your heart at rest. Your doctor can then compare the active and resting pictures. The comparison may show, for example, that your heart muscle receives adequate blood while at rest but not while exercising, or that it's always "gasping for blood." And if the thallium is not seen in a certain part of the heart either during rest or exercise, chances are you've probably already had a heart attack affecting that part of the heart.

Cardiac Catheterization

This is the most invasive and hence most dangerous of these tests. Your doctor will watch as a special dye flows through your coronary arteries, noting where the flow slows or stops. He or she will also "see" the structure of your left ventricle and how it works.

Because catheterization is so potentially dangerous, it will be important that you are carefully screened. A thorough examination performed by a cardiologist will ensure that you are able to withstand the procedure. Tell the doctor about any drugs and/or supplements you are taking, as well as any allergies you may have. (It's a good idea to bring all your medicines and supplements with you to the examination.)

The day of your catheterization, you'll be brought to the hospital's catheterization laboratory, a high-tech area with heart monitors,

X rays, television screens and other devices. After you've been given a sedative, a local anesthetic has been applied to the incision site and an IV line has been started, the doctor will make a small incision in your groin or arm. Then an artery or vein will be opened and a catheter fed into your blood vessel.

Working very carefully, the doctor will push the catheter through your blood vessels toward the heart, guided by "real time" X-ray images tracking the catheter's progress. When the catheter has been threaded up to the target area, a special dye will be injected through the catheter into your bloodstream. Watching the dye flowing through your blood vessels on the screen, the doctor can see any blockage in the coronary arteries, and gather other useful information. (You may feel slightly nauseated, warm or flushed as the dye is injected, and your heart may beat irregularly.)

Cardiac catheterization takes an hour or two, with the catheter actually inside your body for twenty to forty minutes. Afterwards, you'll be bandaged and pressure may be applied to the incision site for several hours to ensure there will be no bleeding. You'll rest for several hours, and your vital signs will be checked regularly. If all goes well, you'll feel fine in a day or two, and the bruise at the incision site will heal in a couple of weeks. Potential side effects include an allergic reaction to the dye, low blood pressure, infections, bleeding, irregular heartbeat, blood vessel perforation, heart attack and stroke.

On the Horizon

Cardiac catheterization and other tests may soon be obsolete, for medical technologists are developing tools that can "see" into the body without cutting or injecting anything into it. For example, ultrafast CT scans combined with cutting-edge computer technology are rapidly making it possible for doctors to see plaque buildups in your coronary arteries and gauge the degree of blockage, if any.

INTERVENTIONAL CARDIOLOGY PROCEDURES AND SURGERY TO TREAT CORONARY HEART DISEASE

Doctors have several medications for combating coronary heart disease, including drugs to thin the blood, lower cholesterol, calm the heart, reduce blood pressure and widen the coronary arteries. If these

Women and Heart Disease

Women don't have to worry too much about heart disease, right? Wrong.

Coronary heart disease, the process that triggers heart attacks, is the single biggest killer of American women. It's true that heart attacks are a big worry for men, starting in their forties, but women face an increasing risk as they go through menopause. It's felt that the "female hormone" estrogen helps shield women from heart disease. When estrogen levels drop during menopause, the shield is lowered. Estrogen replacement therapy can help to continue protecting women from heart disease, but taking estrogen may also raise the risk of breast and uterine cancer.

Woman who are struck by heart attacks tend to fare worse than men, statistically speaking. Only 56 percent of women suffering a heart attack can expect to live another year, compared to 73 percent of male victims. And 31 percent of women who have an attack will likely have a second one within six years, as opposed to 27 percent of the men.

Adding insult to injury, even if they've had bypass surgery, women are more likely than men to die of heart disease, and to fare poorly after angioplasty. We don't know exactly why this is, but it may be partially due to the fact that women tend to be older than men when they undergo the surgery. They may also be sicker, in part because women—and their doctors—are often less tuned in to the risk of heart disease in women.

Beware the special risks: women with diabetes are stricken with heart attacks at twice the rate of nondiabetic women of the same age. The combination of oral contraceptives and smoking is another uniquely female risk factor. Women who smoke and use "the pill" are more likely to be hit with a heart attack or stroke than women who don't smoke or don't use the pill.

don't work, and if there isn't time to wait for dietary and lifestyle changes to reduce the risk of heart disease, interventional cardiology procedures or surgery may be recommended.

Let's take a quick look at the common interventional cardiology procedures for coronary heart disease—angioplasty, stents, atherectomy—as well as coronary artery bypass surgery.

What's the Difference?

Briefly speaking, surgeries are performed by surgeons and interventional cardiology procedures by cardiologists. From the patient's point of view, the distinction is that surgery requires a "big cut" in the body, while interventional cardiology is performed with a catheter pushed through a small incision. As techniques are refined, the distinction may, for all practical purposes, disappear.

Angioplasty: "Ballooning" Away the Blockage

If the coronary artery blockage isn't severe enough to warrant bypass surgery, or if you're not a good candidate for surgery, your physician may suggest percutaneous transluminal coronary angioplasty, otherwise known as coronary angioplasty or simply angioplasty. The idea behind angioplasty is simple: insert a balloon into the partially clogged artery, then inflate the balloon so that it presses against the plaque, compressing it against the artery walls. Whether or not you're a good candidate for angioplasty depends on the size and location of the blockage, whether or not it's heavily calcified (filled with calcium), and your general health.

The procedure usually takes place in the hospital's catheterization laboratory. A small incision is made in the skin near your groin, or on your arm or wrist. Next, the doctor uses a special needle to puncture the target artery, and a thin catheter (tube) is inserted into the artery and threaded up to the blocked coronary artery. A special dye that can be seen on an X ray is injected through the tube to help the doctor precisely locate the blockage. Finally, a balloon-tipped catheter is inserted into the catheter and gently pushed up to the blockage. Once it's there, the balloon is inflated and deflated several times and the plaque is "scrunched" against the artery wall.

You will probably remain in the hospital overnight following your angioplasty as the doctors monitor you, making sure that all went well.

Balloon angioplasty does not cure coronary artery disease. The plaque is still there, and the plaque-building process continues. In 20 to 30 percent of cases, the treated artery will become reblocked within six months. However, angioplasty does buy you time. It keeps the blood flowing and keeps you alive while you change your diet and make the other lifestyle changes necessary to stop the disease process. Of course, there are risks to the procedure. Between 3 and 5 percent of angioplasty patients will suffer a nonfatal heart attack during the procedure, and 2 to 4 percent have to have coronary artery bypass surgery immediately after the angioplasty. One or 2 percent of all the people who undergo angioplasty die as a result of the procedure. Angioplasty is less risky than bypass surgery and requires a shorter recovery period, but should not be undertaken lightly.

Stents: Propping Up Trouble Areas

Knowing that simply "clearing out" clogged arteries is not always enough, physicians will sometimes use special "structural supports" to keep the arteries open. Called coronary stents, these metal coils or mesh tubes are inserted into the artery after angioplasty has widened the opening.

The procedure for inserting a stent is very similar to that of angioplasty, and is sometimes done right after the balloon has been used to "push open" the blocked artery. The stent, which remains in place permanently, reduces the odds of re-blockage.

Atherectomy: Cutting Away the Debris

Angioplasty may not be effective if the "plaque dam" contains calcium, because the balloon doesn't work well enough against calcium-laden plaque. So, instead of trying to "squeeze" the plaque, doctors may try to cut it away with atherectomy.

The preparation for atherectomy is very similar to that for angioplasty or stents. But instead of threading a balloon-tipped catheter into the target coronary artery, doctors will use a catheter with either a rotating burr or a special cutting blade on its end.

Spinning up to 200,000 revolutions per minute, the rotating burr breaks tiny pieces of plaque off the "dam." These float away in the bloodstream, and are eventually cleared away by the body's normal cleansing processes. This approach is called rotational atherectomy. Potential side effects include a temporary slowdown of blood flow and heat damage to the artery wall, plus those seen with angioplasty.

The cutting blade, on the other hand, doesn't throw tiny, disposable pieces of plaque into the bloodstream. Instead, spinning 2,000 times per minute, it shaves off pieces of plaque and immediately draws them into the catheter. When the catheter is pulled out of the body, it takes the tiny pieces of plaque with it. This "slicing" technique is called directional atherectomy. The side effects seen with directional atherectomy are similar to those seen with balloon angioplasty.

Whether rotating or directional, atherectomy takes one to three hours.

Coronary Artery Bypass Surgery: Building a New Road Around the Jam

The theory is simple: if one or more coronary arteries are too clogged up to be useful, divert the blood flow around them. Bypass surgery is a major operation; it may last five or six hours, and you'll likely remain in the hospital's intensive care unit for several days to recover.

The surgery proper begins when the surgeon cuts open your chest. Next, he or she "cracks" your breastbone from top to bottom, pushing the two breastbone "halves" and attached ribs to the side. Ice water is placed on the heart to cool it, then various tubes are used to divert your blood flow away from your heart into a heart-lung machine, where it's oxygenated and returned to the body. The surgeon clamps off the aorta, and the preparation is complete.

Now it's time for the graft, for the bypass itself. Either a vein from your leg, or one already attached to a branch of your aorta, one normally used to nourish the chest wall that can be spared, is used. If a leg vein is used, it is cut out of the leg, sewed onto the aorta, then attached to the blocked coronary artery "downstream" of the blockage. If an artery coming off a branch of your aorta is used, the end coming out of the aorta branch is left in place. The other end is cut away from its attachment and sewn onto the dammed-up coronary artery. The impassable area has been bypassed, your heart muscle can now receive the blood it needs.

All that's left is "cleanup." You are taken off the heart-lung machine and your heart takes over the job of circulating your blood. The surgeon uses stainless steel wires to "sew" your breastbone back together, and your skin is sewn shut.

When you wake up in the intensive care unit after the surgery, you'll probably feel uncomfortable, possibly disoriented and thirsty, groggy, cold and in pain. You'll be hooked up to IVs and monitoring devices. Take heart: most people recover relatively quickly from bypass surgery. If all goes well, you'll be sitting up in a chair a day or two after the surgery, and walking the day after that. You'll be moved out of intensive care within a few days, remaining in the hospital for less than a week as you undergo therapy to clear fluid from your lungs and regain your strength. Various tests will be conducted regularly to monitor your progress.

Coronary artery bypass is most likely to help angina patients who have already made dietary and lifestyle changes, tried the various cholesterol-lowering medications, and have no other health problems that would make the surgery dangerous. Bypass surgery offers dramatic hope but is fraught with danger. "Ideal" candidates have a 1 percent chance of dying during surgery, and a 5 percent risk of suffering a heart attack or other heart damage while under the knife. Overall, some 85 percent of patients do well or very well after bypass. In larger hospitals, the surgery is becoming routine; no one gets excited anymore to hear that a patient has just had a quadruple bypass. Of course, *any* surgery carries risks. There is a small risk of infection, lung and bleeding problems, nerve injury, suffering a heart attack or stroke, or dying during the surgery.

A BRIGHT FUTURE

I'VE COVERED A LOT of material in this book, discussing the "hows" and "whys" of the syndrome I named back in 1988. I've asked you to reassess your thinking on diet and to make small but significant changes in your habits. It all boils down to these basic ideas:

Due to a combination of genetics and lifestyle, many of us are insulin resistant. That is, certain cells in our body don't respond efficiently to insulin's call to accept glucose from the blood. Our pancreas then pumps out extra insulin to correct this problem. Ironically, in doing so it lays the groundwork for another, equally dangerous problem: Syndrome X, which is caused by the combination of insulin resistance plus compensatory hyperinsulinemia.

The cluster of problems that make up Syndrome X—including elevated triglycerides, low HDL cholesterol and smaller, denser LDL particles—encourages damage to the coronary arteries that can trigger a heart attack. The best way to solve this problem is to attack it at the root; that is, to keep insulin levels under control.

The most unique part of this program is a diet that flies in the face of current medical "wisdom," which recommends a high-carbohydrate, low-fat diet for just about everyone. That's good advice for many, but if you have Syndrome X, that diet could be the worst thing for you. Instead, you need to cut *back* on the carbohydrates that lead to increased insulin levels. And you don't want to replace these carbohydrates with protein, for protein also raises insulin. Thus, fat must take the place of some of the carbohydrate in your diet. But not any fat will do. Eating saturated fat pushes up your LDL "bad" cholesterol levels, a problem for all people, whether they have Syndrome X or not. Instead, the carbohydrate should be replaced with unsaturated fat. Thus, with the Syndrome X Diet you get 15 percent of your calories from protein, 40 percent from primarily unsaturated fat and 45 percent from carbohydrate. This 15:40:45 ratio is the key. And it's not just for those with the syndrome. The diet—and the rest of the program—can be helpful for those with elevated LDL cholesterol and other risk factors for heart disease.

Exercise and weight loss complement and strengthen the program, as do the other lifestyle changes. And if they don't do the trick, there are many medicines to help.

After three decades of research into Syndrome X, testing our theories in the laboratory and offering our findings to the medical community for scrutiny and comment, I'm ready to present my ideas to you. I urge you to see your physician to find out whether you have the syndrome and, if you do, follow the simple plan I've outlined in this book to safeguard your health.

Armed with knowledge and a practical plan for treatment, we can begin to conquer Syndrome X and live longer, healthier lives.

PART III

Syndrome X
Menu Plans

TAILORING THE

SYNDROME X DIET ™

THE SYNDROME X DIET™ is designed to provide all the nutrients and calories you need, no matter what size you may be. Naturally, this means it must be flexible, able to expand or shrink enough to accommodate the needs of a 6-foot 2-inch athlete or a 4-foot 10-inch couch potato. Thus, I have devised the baseline 1,200 calorie per day Syndrome X Diet to act as a starting point for everybody. Each of the following menus yields one serving. For most adults, following the 1,200 calorie diet in Chapter 15 will bring about weight loss. If you need to lose weight, and you can manage on 1,200 calories without feeling unduly deprived, then that's where you should begin.

If you don't need to lose weight, or if your caloric needs exceed 1,200 calories, there are a couple of ways to adapt this diet. In Chapter 17, you'll find recipes for snacks that provide 100, 200 or 300 calories, in the proper Syndrome X Diet ratio of 15 percent protein, 40 percent fat and 45 percent carbohydrate. By adding these snacks to your 1,200 calorie diet, you can increase your food intake without worrying about increasing your insulin levels. For example, if you need a 1,500 calorie diet per day, follow the 1,200 calorie diet and add in 300 calories' worth of designated snacks.

You may also proportionately increase the serving size of all items listed in the diet to make up your calorie deficit. For example, if you eat one and a quarter times the amount of food on the baseline diet, you'll take in 1,500 calories per day. If you need 1,500 calories per day, just increase the portions listed for the 1,200 calorie diet by one-fourth (i.e., 4 ounces of meat becomes 5 ounces, 1 cup becomes 1¼ cups). Remember: if you increase the serving size of one item at a meal, the serving sizes of all other items at that meal must also be increased to keep the protein/fat/carbohydrate ratio intact. If you need a 2,400 calorie diet, you can simply double the portions of the 1,200 calorie diet.

Chapter 16 contains the 1,800 calorie version of the Syndrome X Diet, a typical maintenance level for many people. Like the 1,200 calorie diet, it can be adjusted to suit your needs by adding snacks or increasing portions. If you want to adapt the diet to include your own food preferences, try switching menu items from the same category, as long as each item has the same number of calories and proportions of fat, protein and carbohydrate. For example, a ½ cup serving of green peas can be exchanged for 1⅓ cups of green beans.

Cooking won't be a problem on either the 1,200 or 1,800 Syndrome X diets, for most dishes in the meal plans are standard. I have provided cooking instructions only when necessary.

A word about alcohol: remember that alcoholic beverages contain calories that need to be factored into your calorie count. For example, an average "light" beer contains approximately 100 calories, and a standard beer contains 150 calories. A glass of red or white wine has approximately 75 calories, a piña colada boasts 525 calories, and a gin and tonic roughly 170. Different alcoholic beverages contain different amounts of carbohydrates. If you are consuming only a few drinks per day, this should not prove to be a major hurdle to maintaining the 15:40:45 ratio. In general, it is best to avoid drinks rich in carbohydrates, like calorie-laden piña coladas, and stick to simple drinks. However, an occasional "sin" is easily forgiven. It's the daily pattern, over the long haul, that's crucial.

Now, get ready for a lifetime of good eating and good health!

MENU PLANS FOR THE

1,200 CALORIE DIET

DAY 1

Breakfast

	Saturated Calories	Mono & Poly Calories	Protein Calories	Carb Calories	Total Calories	Cholesterol (mg)
½ cup cooked oatmeal with cinnamon	0	11	11	51	73	0
1½ tsp. safflower margarine	4	44	0	0	48	0
topped with 1 tsp. sliced almonds	1	12	1	2	16	0
⅓ cup low-fat milk	2	3	11	18	34	3
½ small grapefruit	0	1	1	30	32	0
1 thin slice Canadian bacon	5	9	13	3	30	9
Noncaloric beverage	0	0	0	0	0	0
TOTALS	12	80	37	104	233	12
Total proportions	5%	34.5%	15.5%	45%		

Note: Each menu yields 1 serving.

	Saturated Calories	Mono & Poly Calories	Protein Calories	Carb Calories	Total Calories	Cholesterol (mg)
Lunch						
Peanut butter sandwich special:						
4 tsp. peanut butter	27	71	17	12	127	0
½ tsp. toasted sesame seeds	0	5	2	1	8	0
2 tsp. honey	0	0	0	43	43	0
¼ cup green seedless grapes cut in halves	0	0	0	12	12	0
on 5 toasted bread rounds (crackers)	0	10	14	68	92	0
Green salad with 1 cup lettuce	0	0	1	7	8	0
6 tomato wedges	0	0	0	18	18	0
cucumber slices	0	0	0	2	2	0
1½ Tbsp. cooked shrimp	1	4	22	1	28	49
1½ tsp. vinaigrette	0	31	0	0	31	0
Noncaloric beverage	0	0	0	0	0	0
TOTALS	28	121	56	164	369	49
Total proportions	8%	32%	15%	45%		
Dinner						
1.6 oz. roasted turkey breast with no skin	4	11	61	0	76	33
3 Tbsp. cranberry sauce	0	0	4	75	79	0
¾ cup mashed potatoes	8	29	6	117	160	2
with 1 generous tsp. safflower margarine	8	70	0	0	78	0
¼ baked yam with 2 tsp. safflower margarine	7	64	2	34	107	3
½ cup fresh peas	0	3	16	46	65	0
with 1 tsp. safflower margarine	4	39	0	0	43	0
Noncaloric beverage	0	0	0	0	0	0
TOTALS	31	216	89	272	608	38
Total proportions	5%	35%	15%	45%		

DAY 2

Breakfast

	Saturated Calories	Mono & Poly Calories	Protein Calories	Carb Calories	Total Calories	Cholesterol (mg)
4 oz. fresh orange juice	0	0	3	52	55	0
½ oat bran English muffin	0	6	9	53	68	0
with 1½ tsp. safflower margarine	5	45	0	0	50	0
1 oz. turkey sausage	13	23	24	0	60	23
Noncaloric beverage	0	0	0	0	0	0
TOTALS	18	74	36	105	233	23
Total proportions	8%	32%	15%	45%		

Lunch

	Saturated Calories	Mono & Poly Calories	Protein Calories	Carb Calories	Total Calories	Cholesterol (mg)
Open-faced Turkey Waldorf sandwich: 2 oz. diced turkey	5	7	44	2	58	20
with 4 tsp. safflower mayo	9	113	3	5	130	0
chopped celery	1	8	1	1	11	0
1 chopped walnut half, apple and lemon juice on 1 slice thin wheat toast	0	9	9	46	64	0
1 cup grapes	0	0	1	63	64	0
2 dried dates	0	0	1	49	50	0
Noncaloric beverage	0	0	0	0	0	0
TOTALS	15	137	59	166	377	20
Total proportions	4%	36%	15%	45%		

Dinner

	Saturated Calories	Mono & Poly Calories	Protein Calories	Carb Calories	Total Calories	Cholesterol (mg)
Chick-peas, sausage and spinach: ⅔ cup cooked chick-peas	3	36	57	181	277	0
with ¼ cup onion and ½ tsp. cinnamon	0	1	2	12	15	0
1 small fresh or canned tomato	0	0	3	15	18	0
⅔ cup fresh spinach (packed)	0	0	4	5	9	0
2 Tbsp. golden raisins	0	0	2	57	59	0

	Saturated Calories	Mono & Poly Calories	Protein Calories	Carb Calories	Total Calories	Cholesterol (mg)
sautéed in olive oil with spices to taste	12	77	0	0	89	0
1 small link Italian sausage	42	72	25	1	140	34
Noncaloric beverage	0	0	0	0	0	0
TOTALS	57	186	93	271	607	34
Total proportions	9%	31%	15%	45%		

DAY 3

Breakfast

	Saturated Calories	Mono & Poly Calories	Protein Calories	Carb Calories	Total Calories	Cholesterol (mg)
½ cup raisin bran dry cereal	0	4	10	62	76	0
with ¼ cup low-fat milk	1	2	8	14	25	2
1 small slice Canadian bacon	5	8	13	3	29	9
½ slice rye toast	0	4	5	26	35	0
with 2 tsp. safflower margarine	7	61	0	0	68	0
Noncaloric beverage	0	0	0	0	0	0
TOTALS	13	79	36	105	233	11
Total proportions	6%	34%	15%	45%		

Lunch

	Saturated Calories	Mono & Poly Calories	Protein Calories	Carb Calories	Total Calories	Cholesterol (mg)
Ham and coleslaw sandwich: 2 oz. sliced cured ham	7	23	41	0	71	22
layered with ⅔ cup shredded cabbage	0	0	2	7	9	0
mixed with 3½ tsp. safflower mayo	8	97	3	6	114	0
open-faced on 1 slice pumpernickel bread	0	7	10	62	79	0
1 generous cup fresh pineapple	0	6	1	91	98	0
Noncaloric beverage	0	0	0	0	0	0
TOTALS	15	133	57	166	371	22
Total proportions	4%	36%	16%	44%		

	Saturated Calories	Mono & Poly Calories	Protein Calories	Carb Calories	Total Calories	Cholesterol (mg)
Dinner						
Tuna kebabs:						
2 oz. fresh tuna broiled	7	19	53	0	79	21
with 4 cherry tomatoes	0	1	1	10	12	0
and ½ cup eggplant	0	0	1	10	11	0
drizzled with scant 2 tsp. garlic olive oil with vinegar and oregano	8	65	0	0	73	0
over ⅔ cup cooked rice	0	1	12	137	150	0
1 cup lettuce and spinach salad with a sprinkle of Canadian bacon bits	3	6	14	7	30	7
and 1 Tbsp. vinaigrette	10	72	1	2	85	0
1 medium sourdough roll	0	7	8	93	108	0
½ cup summer squash	0	0	1	12	13	0
stir-fried in 1 tsp. olive oil	5	38	0	0	43	0
Noncaloric beverage	0	0	0	0	0	0
TOTALS	33	209	91	271	604	28
Total proportions	5%	35%	15%	45%		

DAY 4

Breakfast

	Saturated Calories	Mono & Poly Calories	Protein Calories	Carb Calories	Total Calories	Cholesterol (mg)
⅓ cup cooked cream of wheat	0	1	6	39	46	0
with 1 tsp. safflower margarine	3	34	0	0	37	0
⅔ cup fresh strawberries	0	0	2	29	31	0
½ slice whole wheat toast	0	6	7	31	44	0
with 1½ generous tsp. safflower margarine	4	43	0	0	47	0
Scant 3 Tbsp. low-fat cottage cheese	3	2	21	6	32	3
Noncaloric beverage	0	0	0	0	0	0
TOTALS	10	86	36	105	237	3
Total proportions	4%	36%	15%	45%		

	Saturated Calories	Mono & Poly Calories	Protein Calories	Carb Calories	Total Calories	Cholesterol (mg)
Lunch						
Chicken Dijon salad sandwich:						
1.3 oz. white-meat chicken	3	7	47	7	64	32
4 tsp. safflower mayo	10	114	3	5	132	0
½ tsp. Dijon mustard	0	0	0	2	2	0
green onions, dill	0	0	0	2	2	0
1 lettuce leaf	0	0	0	2	2	0
2 slices tomato	0	0	0	7	7	0
open-faced on 1 slice French bread	0	11	8	62	81	0
1 small fresh pear	0	1	1	80	82	0
Noncaloric beverage	0	0	0	0	0	0
TOTALS	13	133	59	167	372	32
Total proportions	4%	36%	15%	45%		
Dinner						
3.5 oz. corned beef with fat cut off	25	102	64	2	193	87
⅓ cup cooked cabbage	0	1	2	9	12	0
⅓ cup cooked carrots with 1 tsp. safflower margarine	0	1	3	22	26	0
	3	34	0	0	37	0
⅔ boiled potato with 1½ tsp. safflower margarine	0	1	6	72	79	0
	5	45	0	0	50	0
3 Tbsp. cooked onion	0	1	1	9	11	0
⅓ cup cooked celery	0	0	1	7	8	0
1 sliver carrot cake	0	24	13	96	133	0
with 5 tsp. glaze frosting	0	0	0	54	54	0
Noncaloric beverage	0	0	0	0	0	0
TOTALS	33	209	90	271	603	87
Total proportions	5%	35%	15%	45%		

	Saturated Calories	Mono & Poly Calories	Protein Calories	Carb Calories	Total Calories	Cholesterol (mg)

DAY 5

Breakfast

	Saturated Calories	Mono & Poly Calories	Protein Calories	Carb Calories	Total Calories	Cholesterol (mg)
4 large stewed prunes	0	0	3	79	82	0
topped with ½ tsp. safflower margarine	1	15	0	0	16	0
1 oz. turkey sausage	13	22	27	0	62	23
½ slice rye toast	0	4	5	26	35	0
with 1 tsp. safflower margarine	3	34	0	0	37	0
Noncaloric beverage	0	0	0	0	0	0
TOTALS	17	75	35	105	232	23
Total proportions	7%	33%	15%	45%		

Lunch

	Saturated Calories	Mono & Poly Calories	Protein Calories	Carb Calories	Total Calories	Cholesterol (mg)
Vegetable stew:						
⅓ cup sweet potato	0	0	3	37	40	0
sautéed with 2 tsp. onion	0	0	0	2	2	0
½ cup zucchini	0	1	2	12	15	0
¼ cup red bell pepper	0	1	1	5	7	0
¼ cup baby lima beans	0	1	14	40	55	0
⅓ cup green beans	0	1	3	13	17	0
½ tsp. curry powder, dash saffron, salt, and other spices to taste and 2 tsp. olive oil	9	71	0	0	80	0
1 small slice toasted French bread	0	5	8	53	66	0
brushed with 1 tsp. garlic olive oil	5	35	0	0	40	0
and 3 Tbsp. diced tomato marinated in scant	0	0	1	7	8	0
1 tsp. balsamic vinaigrette	1	7	0	0	8	0
1 oz. fresh grilled tuna	2	10	28	0	40	11
Noncaloric beverage	0	0	0	0	0	0
TOTALS	17	132	60	169	378	11
Total proportions	4%	36%	15%	45%		

	Saturated Calories	Mono & Poly Calories	Protein Calories	Carb Calories	Total Calories	Cholesterol (mg)

Dinner

	Saturated Calories	Mono & Poly Calories	Protein Calories	Carb Calories	Total Calories	Cholesterol (mg)
²/₃ cup gazpacho	1	12	1	23	37	0
1 chicken enchilada with 1 oz. white meat in red sauce and salsa	10	101	48	65	224	28
Generous ¹/₂ cup cooked rice	0	1	10	115	126	0
¹/₃ cup refried beans	3	6	21	58	88	0
with scant 1¹/₂ tsp. olive oil	6	49	0	0	55	0
1 cup green salad with a few bacon bits	0	0	9	8	17	0
and 2 tsp. oil and vinegar dressing	9	40	0	1	50	28
Noncaloric beverage	0	0	0	0	0	0
TOTALS	29	209	89	270	597	56
Total proportions	5%	35%	15%	45%		

DAY 6

Breakfast

	Saturated Calories	Mono & Poly Calories	Protein Calories	Carb Calories	Total Calories	Cholesterol (mg)
1 small toasted bagel	0	11	15	70	96	0
with 2 tsp. safflower margarine	7	61	0	0	68	0
²/₃ cup low-fat milk	5	7	21	35	68	6
Noncaloric beverage	0	0	0	0	0	0
TOTALS	12	79	36	105	232	6
Dietary proportions	5%	35%	15%	45%		

Lunch

	Saturated Calories	Mono & Poly Calories	Protein Calories	Carb Calories	Total Calories	Cholesterol (mg)
♦ Greek tofu spinach pie: whole wheat crust	0	5	9	64	78	0
oil, garlic, salt, lemon juice	8	89	0	0	97	0
minced onion	0	0	1	4	5	0
firm tofu	7	18	34	8	67	0
fresh cooked spinach	0	0	2	3	5	0
Greek olives	0	12	0	9	21	0
1 sourdough roll	0	8	12	78	98	0

	Saturated Calories	Mono & Poly Calories	Protein Calories	Carb Calories	Total Calories	Cholesterol (mg)
Noncaloric beverage	0	0	0	0	0	0
TOTALS	15	132	58	166	371	0
Total proportions	4%	36%	15%	45%		

♦ The ingredients listed above represent one serving or one-eighth of the pie. The recipe below makes a whole pie.

Preheat oven to 350°. Use a 9-inch whole wheat piecrust, made with canola or safflower oil, which you can make or purchase.

To prepare the filling, in a large bowl mix 4 scant tablespoons safflower oil, 1 teaspoon minced garlic or garlic powder, 2 teaspoons salt, 2 tablespoons fresh lemon juice and 12 chopped Greek olives. Add 1 pound very firm and crumbled tofu. Set it aside to marinate.

Sauté 2 tablespoons olive oil and 1 cup minced onion until the onion is slightly burnt. Add 3 cups fresh chopped spinach. Sauté 2½ minutes. Add to the tofu mixture. Transfer into the prebaked piecrust and spread out evenly, firming the mixture level. Bake for 30 minutes at 350°.

Dinner

	Saturated Calories	Mono & Poly Calories	Protein Calories	Carb Calories	Total Calories	Cholesterol (mg)
Lamb fondue:						
1.5 oz. lamb with fat trimmed	15	12	51	0	78	0
1 tsp. safflower oil (residue from cooking lamb)	3	37	0	0	40	0
⅔ cup rice pilaf	0	1	11	133	145	0
with 3 Tbsp. onion	0	0	1	9	10	0
and scant ½ tsp. safflower margarine	5	41	0	0	46	0
Dipping sauces for lamb:						
4 tsp. yogurt chutney	7	4	5	3	19	0
4 tsp. dill chutney mixed with 1 Tbsp. safflower oil and Dijon mustard to taste	7	78	2	3	90	0
⅓ cup brussels sprouts	1	2	5	19	27	0
⅔ artichoke dipped in lemon juice	0	2	7	34	43	0
1 sliver carrot cake, unfrosted	8	21	8	70	107	0

	Saturated Calories	Mono & Poly Calories	Protein Calories	Carb Calories	Total Calories	Cholesterol (mg)
Noncaloric beverage	0	0	0	0	0	0
TOTALS	46	198	90	271	605	0
Total proportions	8%	32%	15%	45%		

DAY 7

Breakfast

	Saturated Calories	Mono & Poly Calories	Protein Calories	Carb Calories	Total Calories	Cholesterol (mg)
⅔ cup melon balls	0	1	3	34	38	0
1 5-in. buttermilk pancake	1	3	9	71	84	0
with 1½ tsp. safflower margarine	5	45	0	0	50	0
1 generous oz. chicken apple sausage	13	25	24	0	62	25
Noncaloric beverage	0	0	0	0	0	0
TOTALS	19	74	36	105	234	25
Total proportions	8%	32%	15%	45%		

Lunch

	Saturated Calories	Mono & Poly Calories	Protein Calories	Carb Calories	Total Calories	Cholesterol (mg)
Open-faced Waldorf sandwich: 2 oz. diced turkey	5	7	45	1	58	20
4 tsp. safflower mayo	9	113	3	5	130	0
chopped celery, 1 chopped walnut half, apple and lemon juice	1	8	1	1	11	0
on 1 slice whole wheat toast	0	9	8	48	65	0
1 cup grapes	0	0	1	63	64	0
2 dried dates	0	0	1	49	50	0
Noncaloric beverage	0	0	0	0	0	0
TOTALS	15	137	59	167	378	20
Total proportions	4%	36%	15%	45%		

	Saturated Calories	Mono & Poly Calories	Protein Calories	Carb Calories	Total Calories	Cholesterol (mg)
Dinner						
♦ Tuna sauce spaghetti:						
⅓ cup canned tomatoes with juice	0	1	2	22	25	0
garlic, 1 Tbsp. parsley	0	0	0	1	1	0
2 tsp. olive oil	13	85	0	0	98	0
2 oz. fresh or canned tuna with spices to taste	7	19	53	0	79	21
served over 2 oz. spaghetti	0	10	29	170	209	0
1 small slice garlic bread	0	6	9	32	47	0
with 2 tsp. safflower margarine	7	61	0	0	68	0
1 cup mixed baby greens	0	0	0	2	2	0
with 1½ tsp. vinaigrette	6	26	0	1	33	0
Scant ½ cup black grapes	1	2	1	47	51	0
Noncaloric beverage	0	0	0	0	0	0
TOTALS	34	210	94	275	613	21
Total proportions	6%	34%	15%	45%		

♦ For spaghetti, amounts listed above are for a single serving. Increase ingredients proportionately according to number of 1,200 calorie servings you wish to prepare.

DAY 8

Breakfast

	Saturated Calories	Mono & Poly Calories	Protein Calories	Carb Calories	Total Calories	Cholesterol (mg)
½ cup cooked oatmeal with cinnamon	0	11	11	51	73	0
1½ tsp. safflower margarine	4	44	0	0	48	0
topped with 1½ tsp. sliced almonds	1	12	1	2	16	0
⅓ cup low-fat milk	2	3	11	18	34	3
½ small grapefruit	0	1	1	30	32	0
1 thin slice Canadian bacon	5	9	13	3	30	9
Noncaloric beverage	0	0	0	0	0	0
TOTALS	12	80	37	104	233	12
Total proportions	5%	34.5%	15.5%	45%		

	Saturated Calories	Mono & Poly Calories	Protein Calories	Carb Calories	Total Calories	Cholesterol (mg)
Lunch						
Lamb burger: 1.5 oz. grilled lean lamb patty	12	11	40	0	63	0
with 1 tsp. mustard	0	1	1	2	4	0
and 2 tsp. catsup	0	1	1	9	11	0
on a hamburger roll	0	20	9	82	111	0
2 cucumber slices	0	0	1	4	5	0
⅔ medium tomato drizzled with scant 1 Tbsp. vinaigrette	0	3	3	22	28	0
	0	68	0	1	69	0
5 Greek olives	3	28	1	2	34	0
4 radishes	0	1	1	2	4	0
½ medium to large banana	1	3	2	51	57	0
Noncaloric beverage	0	0	0	0	0	0
TOTALS	16	136	59	175	386	0
Total proportions	4%	35.3%	15.3%	45.4%		
Dinner						
⅔ cup lentil soup topped with 2 tsp. yogurt	6	13	26	65	110	7
2.3 oz. lean ham	9	24	49	0	82	24
1 small baked potato	0	1	11	136	148	0
with 2 tsp. safflower margarine	7	61	0	0	68	0
2 cups green salad with red onions, 4 tsp. feta cheese, 3 tomato slices drizzled with 4 tsp. oil and vinegar dressing	30	85	5	7	127	8
⅔ minted fresh pear poached in grapefruit juice	0	4	1	67	72	0
Noncaloric beverage	0	0	0	0	0	0
TOTALS	52	188	92	275	607	39
Total proportions	9%	31%	15%	45%		

	Saturated Calories	Mono & Poly Calories	Protein Calories	Carb Calories	Total Calories	Cholesterol (mg)
DAY 9						
Breakfast						
4 oz. fresh orange juice	0	0	3	52	55	0
½ oat bran English muffin with 1½ tsp. safflower	0	6	9	53	68	0
margarine	5	45	0	0	50	0
1 oz. turkey sausage	13	23	24	0	60	23
Noncaloric beverage	0	0	0	0	0	0
TOTALS	18	74	36	105	233	23
Total proportions	8%	32%	15%	45%		
Lunch						
Tuna salad pita pocket:						
1.3 oz. fresh or canned light tuna	4	13	36	0	53	14
1 pita pocket	0	8	16	82	106	0
4 tsp. safflower mayo	10	114	3	5	132	0
chopped onion and celery	0	0	0	4	4	0
alfalfa sprouts	0	0	0	1	1	0
1 slice tomato	0	0	1	5	6	0
cucumber slices	0	0	0	1	1	0
⅓ cup mandarin oranges mixed with 4 tsp. vanilla	0	0	1	54	55	0
yogurt	0	3	3	18	24	0
Noncaloric beverage	0	0	0	0	0	0
TOTALS	14	138	60	170	382	14
Total proportions	4%	36%	15%	45%		
Dinner						
1.7 oz lean rib roast beef with fat trimmed	25	35	52	0	112	54
1 baked potato with 1½ tsp. safflower	1	2	17	182	202	0
margarine	5	50	0	0	55	0
1½ cup mixed greens	0	1	4	11	16	0
2 tsp. grated carrot	0	0	0	4	4	0

	Saturated Calories	Mono & Poly Calories	Protein Calories	Carb Calories	Total Calories	Cholesterol (mg)
1/3 tomato cut in wedges	0	1	1	7	9	0
2 tsp. Italian dressing	6	37	0	4	47	0
1 1/2 pieces garlic bread made with 2 tsp. safflower	0	12	16	66	94	0
margarine	7	61	0	0	68	0
Noncaloric beverage	0	0	0	0	0	0
TOTALS	44	199	90	274	607	54
Total proportions	7%	33%	15%	45%		

DAY 10

Breakfast

	Saturated Calories	Mono & Poly Calories	Protein Calories	Carb Calories	Total Calories	Cholesterol (mg)
1/2 cup raisin bran dry cereal	0	4	10	62	76	0
with 1/4 cup low-fat milk	1	2	8	14	25	2
1 small slice Canadian bacon	5	8	13	3	29	9
1/2 slice rye toast	0	4	5	26	35	0
with 2 tsp. safflower margarine	7	61	0	0	68	0
Noncaloric beverage	0	0	0	0	0	0
TOTALS	13	79	36	105	233	11
Total proportions	6%	34%	15%	45%		

Lunch

	Saturated Calories	Mono & Poly Calories	Protein Calories	Carb Calories	Total Calories	Cholesterol (mg)
1 chicken or turkey hot dog	23	49	22	3	97	39
on 1 bun	0	19	14	81	114	0
with 2 tsp. mustard	0	5	3	3	11	0
and 2 tsp. catsup	0	1	1	9	11	0
Generous 1/2 cup sauerkraut	0	1	1	28	30	0
1/2 cup New England clam chowder	13	16	15	30	74	15
with 1/2 tsp. safflower margarine	1	17	0	0	18	0
1 Nabisco chocolate snap cookie	0	0	1	16	17	0
Noncaloric beverage	0	0	0	0	0	0
TOTALS	37	108	57	170	372	54
Total proportions	10%	30%	15%	45%		

	Saturated Calories	Mono & Poly Calories	Protein Calories	Carb Calories	Total Calories	Cholesterol (mg)
Dinner						
2.5 oz. fresh salmon	5	32	55	0	92	40
broiled with 1 tsp. olive oil	6	36	0	0	42	0
½ small baked potato with scant 2 tsp. safflower	0	0	11	100	111	0
margarine	7	58	0	0	65	0
⅔ cup green beans and 2 tsp. olive oil mixed	0	0	5	21	26	0
with lemon juice to taste	7	46	0	0	53	0
1 small sourdough roll with 1 tsp. safflower	0	5	9	53	67	0
margarine	3	34	0	0	37	0
⅔ slice angel food cake	0	0	11	96	107	0
Noncaloric beverage	0	0	0	0	0	0
TOTALS	28	211	91	270	600	40
Total proportions	5%	35%	15%	45%		

DAY 11

Breakfast

	Saturated Calories	Mono & Poly Calories	Protein Calories	Carb Calories	Total Calories	Cholesterol (mg)
⅓ cup cooked cream of wheat	0	1	6	39	46	0
with 1 tsp. safflower margarine	3	34	0	0	37	0
⅔ cup fresh strawberries	0	0	2	29	31	0
½ slice whole wheat toast with 1½ tsp. safflower	0	6	7	31	44	0
margarine	4	43	0	0	47	0
Scant 3 Tbsp. low-fat cottage cheese	3	2	21	6	32	3
Noncaloric beverage	0	0	0	0	0	0
TOTALS	10	86	36	105	237	3
Total proportions	4%	36%	15%	45%		

	Saturated Calories	Mono & Poly Calories	Protein Calories	Carb Calories	Total Calories	Cholesterol (mg)

Lunch

♦ Vegetable tofu burger:						
2 generous tsp. sesame oil	12	82	0	0	94	0
burnt onion, carrot,						
garlic and water chestnuts	0	1	2	9	12	0
1/3 cup chopped fresh						
spinach	0	1	1	3	5	0
1/4 cup firm (not silken) tofu	7	19	34	9	69	0
1 1/2 tsp. toasted sesame						
seeds	2	15	4	1	22	0
on 1 sourdough dinner						
roll (small) or focaccia						
(flatbread)	0	8	12	80	100	0
Fruit salad with 1 small						
fresh peach	0	0	0	32	32	0
and 1/3 banana	0	0	1	33	34	0
Noncaloric beverage	0	0	0	0	0	0
TOTALS	21	126	54	167	368	0
Total proportions	6%	34%	15%	45%		

♦   Preheat oven to 350°. Coat a baking tray with nonstick cooking spray and set aside. Sauté 1 tablespoon minced onion in the sesame oil until slightly burnt. Add 2 teaspoons peeled and grated carrot and sauté for 4 to 5 minutes. Add salt to taste, a pinch of garlic powder, 2 teaspoons chopped water chestnuts and the chopped fresh spinach. Mix and remove from the heat. Using a blender, crumble the tofu. Mix the tofu into the other ingredients and return to the heat. Add the toasted sesame seeds. Form the mixture into a patty. Bake at 350° on the coated tray for 25 minutes, or until golden brown. Serve on a small roll. It's also delicious served on focaccia (flat bread).

Dinner

Generous 1/3 cup chicken,						
cubed	5	15	40	5	65	26
stir-fried in 1 1/2 tsp. canola						
or sesame oil	4	47	0	0	51	0
and rolled in 2 tsp. sesame						
seeds	3	23	5	2	33	0
♦ Udon soup:						
1 to 2 shiitake mushrooms	0	1	2	21	24	0

	Saturated Calories	Mono & Poly Calories	Protein Calories	Carb Calories	Total Calories	Cholesterol (mg)
½ cup green cabbage	0	3	5	19	27	0
⅓ cup spinach or collard greens	0	1	3	5	9	0
1 generous Tbsp. firm tofu, cubed	2	16	15	5	38	0
⅔ cup cooked Udon noodles (thick white noodles)	0	15	17	101	133	34
1½ tsp. tahini	3	42	3	4	52	0
¼ tsp. miso	0	0	1	3	4	0
¼ tsp. tamari sauce	0	0	0	1	1	0
1½ tsp. sesame oil with garlic to taste	5	55	0	0	60	0
pinch onion powder						
fresh ginger						
½ cup strawberry sorbet	0	1	1	102	104	0
Noncaloric beverage	0	0	0	0	0	0
TOTALS	22	219	92	268	601	60
Total proportions	4%	36%	15%	45%		

♦ Place the shiitake mushroom pieces in a pot of cold water. Bring water to a boil, then reduce heat and simmer for 12 minutes. Add cabbage and boil until barely soft. Add spinach and boil another 1 minute until barely wilted and still a bright green color. Drain vegetables immediately into a colander and refresh by rinsing briefly with cold running water. Put 1¼ cups fresh water in the pot and bring to a boil. Turn heat to low and add tofu cubes.

Break the Udon noodles into thirds and cook according to the package instructions. When done, add cooked noodles to the tofu pot.

Whisk thoroughly or blend in a blender ½ cup of the water from the tofu pot and the raw tahini, miso, tamari sauce, and sesame oil with garlic, onion powder and ginger to taste. (Tahini, miso, tamari and Udon noodles are available in grocery stores.) Add to the tofu pot along with the drained mushrooms, spinach and cabbage. Reheat, being careful not to boil the soup. Serve hot.

	Saturated Calories	Mono & Poly Calories	Protein Calories	Carb Calories	Total Calories	Cholesterol (mg)

DAY 12

Breakfast

	Saturated Calories	Mono & Poly Calories	Protein Calories	Carb Calories	Total Calories	Cholesterol (mg)
4 large stewed prunes topped with 1/2 tsp. safflower	0	0	3	79	82	0
margarine	1	15	0	0	16	0
Scant 1 oz. turkey sausage	13	22	27	0	62	23
1/2 slice rye toast with 1 tsp. safflower	0	4	5	26	35	0
margarine	3	34	0	0	37	0
Noncaloric beverage	0	0	0	0	0	0
TOTALS	17	75	35	105	232	23
Total proportions	7%	33%	15%	45%		

Lunch

	Saturated Calories	Mono & Poly Calories	Protein Calories	Carb Calories	Total Calories	Cholesterol (mg)
♦ White bean and cabbage soup with 1/2 cup cooked small white beans	1	2	37	101	141	0
1/3 cup cabbage	0	0	1	4	5	0
1/4 cup celery	0	0	0	3	3	0
scant 1/4 cup carrots	0	0	1	9	10	0
1 Tbsp. onion sautéed in 1 1/2 generous tsp. safflower oil	7	63	0	0	70	0
1/4 cup canned tomatoes	0	5	2	18	25	0
1 Tbsp. lemon juice	0	0	0	2	2	0
1 tsp. brown sugar	0	0	0	11	11	0
2/3 cup chicken broth (more, if needed)	2	4	3	4	13	0
1/4 tsp. caraway seed, thyme, spices to taste	0	1	1	5	7	0
11 dry-roasted almonds	0	60	11	7	78	0
Noncaloric beverage	0	0	0	0	0	0
TOTALS	10	135	56	167	368	0
Total proportions	3%	37%	15%	45%		

♦ Before you make this hearty soup, it is best to soak the beans overnight in cold water and drain before preparing.

	Saturated Calories	Mono & Poly Calories	Protein Calories	Carb Calories	Total Calories	Cholesterol (mg)

Dinner

	Saturated Calories	Mono & Poly Calories	Protein Calories	Carb Calories	Total Calories	Cholesterol (mg)
2.3 oz. lean meat loaf (ground beef)	43	67	64	35	209	72
with 3 Tbsp. onion	0	0	1	8	9	0
sautéed in 1 tsp. safflower margarine	3	34	0	0	37	0
and topped with 2 tsp. tomato sauce	0	1	1	10	12	0
⅓ cup cauliflower	0	1	3	7	11	0
with 1 tsp. safflower margarine	3	34	0	0	37	0
⅔ cup boiled collard greens with lemon juice	0	1	4	13	18	0
and 1 tsp. diced Canadian bacon	1	3	6	0	10	0
⅔ cup new potatoes	1	1	13	135	150	0
with 1½ tsp. olive oil and spices	7	46	0	0	53	0
Scant ⅓ cup strawberry sorbet	0	0	1	64	65	0
Noncaloric beverage	0	0	0	0	0	0
TOTALS	58	188	93	272	611	72
Total proportions	9%	31%	15%	45%		

DAY 13

Breakfast

	Saturated Calories	Mono & Poly Calories	Protein Calories	Carb Calories	Total Calories	Cholesterol (mg)
1 small toasted bagel	0	11	15	70	96	0
with 2 tsp. safflower margarine	7	61	0	0	68	0
⅔ cup low-fat milk	5	7	21	35	68	6
Noncaloric beverage	0	0	0	0	0	0
TOTALS	12	79	36	105	232	6
Total proportions	5%	35%	15%	45%		

Lunch

	Saturated Calories	Mono & Poly Calories	Protein Calories	Carb Calories	Total Calories	Cholesterol (mg)
◆ Hungarian beef stew:						
1.5 oz. lean sirloin	11	19	43	0	73	15
1½ tsp. canola oil	5	50	0	0	55	0
½ clove garlic, spices and						
1 Tbsp. beef broth	0	0	2	1	3	1
2 tsp. onion	0	0	0	2	2	0
1 tsp. balsamic vinegar	0	0	0	0	0	0
½ Romano tomato	0	1	1	9	11	0
⅓ large potato	0	0	4	55	59	0
¼ cup boiled celery root	0	1	1	11	13	0
⅓ cup shredded carrot	0	0	2	21	23	0
⅓ cup cucumber slices	0	0	1	4	5	0
1½ Tbsp. julienne beets	0	0	3	15	18	0
separately marinated in						
vinaigrette (2½ tsp. total)	0	60	0	1	61	0
with 2 tomato wedges	0	1	2	9	12	0
on 1 cup butter lettuce	0	1	1	8	10	0
½ apple	0	0	0	33	33	0
Noncaloric beverage	0	0	0	0	0	0
TOTALS	16	133	60	169	378	16
Total proportions	4%	36%	15%	45%		

◆ Cut the meat into 1-inch cubes. Pat dry with toweling and sprinkle with salt. Put the oil into a skillet. When the pan is hot, brown all sides of the meat, turning frequently. Transfer the meat to a Dutch oven or large pot with a lid. Add beef broth, onion, tomato, garlic and bay leaf. Cover and simmer for 1½ hours or longer, stirring occasionally. Add more beef broth or water as necessary to prevent the stew from burning. Remove bay leaf and garlic clove. Add the cubed potato and simmer another 30 minutes or until potatoes are done. Add the balsamic vinegar and salt to taste. Thicken with 1 teaspoon flour, if desired. Variation: add parsley, carrots and peas.

Dinner

	Saturated Calories	Mono & Poly Calories	Protein Calories	Carb Calories	Total Calories	Cholesterol (mg)
◆ Seared scallops and						
fettuccini:						
2.7 oz. fresh scallops	1	5	52	7	65	25
sautéed in 2 tsp. olive oil						
and ½ tsp. minced garlic	15	104	0	0	119	0

	Saturated Calories	Mono & Poly Calories	Protein Calories	Carb Calories	Total Calories	Cholesterol (mg)
1 tsp. parsley	0	0	0	1	1	0
1½ tsp. dry red pepper flakes (or to taste)	0	0	0	1	1	0
1 tsp. capers and spices to taste	0	0	0	2	2	0
2 oz. fettuccini or spaghetti noodles	0	10	29	172	211	0
1 small slice garlic bread made with 2 tsp. safflower margarine	0 7	6 61	8 0	32 0	46 68	0 0
1 cup mixed baby greens with 1½ tsp. vinaigrette	0 6	0 26	0 0	2 1	2 33	0 0
⅓ small guava	0	1	1	30	32	0
⅔ fresh peach	0	1	1	24	26	0
Noncaloric beverage	0	0	0	0	0	0
TOTALS	29	214	91	272	606	25
Total proportions	5%	35%	15%	45%		

♦ Rinse scallops in cold water and dry gently and thoroughly with toweling. Cut into $3/8$-inch pieces. Put the olive oil and minced garlic into a saucepan and sauté until light golden. Add parsley, hot peppers and capers (optional) and stir. When adding the hot peppers, start with a pinch per serving and add more later, if desired. Turn the heat to high and when hot add the scallops and salt to taste. Cook on high for 1 minute, stirring constantly. When the scallops turn a flat white, remove them from the heat and set aside. Cook the fettuccini or spaghetti noodles until firm (al dente). Turn the heat up high again on the scallops for a few seconds to reheat them. Do not boil away the delicious liquid from the scallops. Serve over drained pasta.

DAY 14

Breakfast

⅔ cup melon balls	0	1	3	34	38	0
1 5-in. buttermilk pancake with 1½ tsp. safflower margarine	1 5	3 45	9 0	71 0	84 50	0 0
1 generous oz. chicken apple sausage	13	25	24	0	62	25

	Saturated Calories	Mono & Poly Calories	Protein Calories	Carb Calories	Total Calories	Cholesterol (mg)
Noncaloric beverage	0	0	0	0	0	0
TOTALS	19	74	36	105	234	25
Total proportions	8%	32%	15%	45%		

Lunch

	Saturated Calories	Mono & Poly Calories	Protein Calories	Carb Calories	Total Calories	Cholesterol (mg)
²/₃ cup black bean soup	2	9	13	53	77	0
4 asparagus spears	1	5	5	11	22	0
wrapped in 1½ slices white-meat turkey drizzled with 2 tsp.	0	3	24	1	28	4
vinaigrette	6	42	0	1	49	0
1½ slices French bread	0	12	14	67	93	0
with 2 tsp. safflower margarine	7	61	0	0	68	0
3 chocolate snap cookies	0	0	2	34	36	0
Noncaloric beverage	0	0	0	0	0	0
TOTALS	16	132	58	167	373	4
Total proportions	4%	36%	15%	45%		

Dinner

	Saturated Calories	Mono & Poly Calories	Protein Calories	Carb Calories	Total Calories	Cholesterol (mg)
♦ Linguini and clams: 1.7 oz. canned clams	1	8	48	10	67	31
2 tsp. olive oil	15	104	0	0	119	0
clove garlic, 1 tsp. parsley, 1 tsp. roasted hot red peppers	0	0	0	2	2	0
2 oz. linguini	0	10	29	171	210	0
1½ generous slices garlic bread	0	13	16	86	115	0
made with 2 tsp. safflower margarine topping	7	61	0	0	68	0
2 cups mixed baby greens	0	0	0	4	4	0
1½ tsp. vinaigrette	5	21	0	1	27	0
Noncaloric beverage	0	0	0	0	0	0
TOTALS	28	217	93	274	612	31
Total proportions	5%	35%	15%	45%		

♦ Drain clams thoroughly and set aside. Put the olive oil and minced garlic into a saucepan and sauté until light golden. Add parsley and a pinch of hot peppers (to taste). Add clams and salt to taste. Sauté for 30 to 40 seconds on medium-high heat. Serve over linguini, cooked firm to the bite (al dente).

	Saturated Calories	Mono & Poly Calories	Protein Calories	Carb Calories	Total Calories	Cholesterol (mg)
DAY 15						
Breakfast						
½ cup cooked oatmeal with cinnamon	0	11	11	51	73	0
1½ tsp. safflower margarine	4	44	0	0	48	0
topped with 1 tsp. sliced almonds	1	12	1	2	16	0
⅓ cup low-fat milk	2	3	11	18	34	3
½ small grapefruit	0	1	1	30	32	0
1 thin slice Canadian bacon	5	9	13	3	30	9
Noncaloric beverage	0	0	0	0	0	0
TOTALS	12	80	37	104	233	12
Total proportions	5%	34.5%	15.5%	45%		
Lunch						
Baked sesame burger:						
⅔ tofu burger (purchased at the grocery)	5	30	30	10	75	0
sprinkled with scant 2 tsp. sunflower seeds	3	20	6	7	36	0
and 1½ tsp. toasted sesame seeds	2	11	3	1	17	0
Alfalfa sprouts	0	0	2	3	5	0
tamari sauce	0	0	0	7	7	0
and 1¼ tsp. tahini dressing	3	25	4	5	37	0
on 1 hamburger bun	0	20	10	82	112	0
1½ cups mixed baby greens	0	0	0	3	3	0
cucumber slices	0	0	0	2	2	0
3 tomato wedges	0	0	0	4	4	0
1½ tsp. raspberry vinaigrette	0	30	0	1	31	0
1 medium fresh fig	0	2	1	40	43	0

	Saturated Calories	Mono & Poly Calories	Protein Calories	Carb Calories	Total Calories	Cholesterol (mg)
Noncaloric beverage	0	0	0	0	0	0
TOTALS	13	138	56	165	372	0
Total proportions	3%	37%	15%	45%		

Dinner

	Saturated Calories	Mono & Poly Calories	Protein Calories	Carb Calories	Total Calories	Cholesterol (mg)
3 oz. lean baked ham	11	24	64	0	99	33
1/3 cup yams	0	1	3	51	55	0
with 1 1/2 tsp. safflower margarine	5	41	0	0	46	0
1/3 cup green beans	0	1	3	14	18	0
1/3 cup brussels sprouts	1	2	6	19	28	0
scant 2 tsp. safflower margarine	6	56	0	0	62	0
Scant 1/3 cup mashed potato	5	15	9	73	102	0
1 sliver apple pie (1/8 of a pie)	14	58	7	115	194	0
Noncaloric beverage	0	0	0	0	0	0
TOTALS	42	198	92	272	604	33
Total proportions	7%	33%	15%	45%		

DAY 16

Breakfast

	Saturated Calories	Mono & Poly Calories	Protein Calories	Carb Calories	Total Calories	Cholesterol (mg)
4 oz. fresh orange juice	0	0	3	52	55	0
1/2 oat bran English muffin	0	6	9	53	68	0
with 1 1/2 generous tsp. safflower margarine	5	45	0	0	50	0
1 oz. turkey sausage	13	23	24	0	60	23
Noncaloric beverage	0	0	0	0	0	0
TOTALS	18	74	36	105	233	23
Total proportions	8%	32%	15%	45%		

	Saturated Calories	Mono & Poly Calories	Protein Calories	Carb Calories	Total Calories	Cholesterol (mg)
Lunch						
1.5 oz. sliced turkey breast	9	29	44	0	82	27
1/3 cup potato salad made with safflower mayo, oil and vinegar	5	63	2	36	106	0
1 1/2 biscuits (from mix)	0	40	11	70	121	0
1 small slice watermelon (2/3 cup)	0	3	3	32	38	0
1/3 oz. jelly beans	0	0	0	31	31	0
Noncaloric beverage	0	0	0	0	0	0
TOTALS	14	135	60	169	378	27
Total proportions	4%	36%	15%	45%		
Dinner						
3.3 oz. fresh crab	1	5	63	2	71	35
dipped in 4 tsp. melted safflower margarine mixed with lemon to taste	13	118	1	1	133	0
1/3 cup cooked spinach	0	1	7	9	17	0
with spices and 1 tsp. safflower margarine	3	34	0	0	37	0
2/3 large baked potato	0	1	14	164	179	0
2 tsp. chives	0	0	0	1	1	0
1 generous tsp. safflower margarine	4	37	0	0	41	0
2-inch square gingerbread (from mix)	0	24	5	95	124	0
Noncaloric beverage	0	0	0	0	0	0
TOTALS	21	220	90	272	603	35
Total proportions	3%	37%	15%	45%		

DAY 17

Breakfast

1/2 cup raisin bran dry cereal	0	4	10	62	76	0
with 1/4 cup low-fat milk	1	2	8	14	25	2

	Saturated Calories	Mono & Poly Calories	Protein Calories	Carb Calories	Total Calories	Cholesterol (mg)
1 small slice Canadian bacon	5	8	13	3	29	9
½ slice rye toast	0	4	5	26	35	0
with 2 tsp. safflower margarine	7	61	0	0	68	0
Noncaloric beverage	0	0	0	0	0	0
TOTALS	13	79	36	105	233	11
Total proportions	6%	34%	15%	45%		

Lunch

Crab sandwich: 1.5 oz. crabmeat	0	1	28	0	29	15
with 3½ generous tsp. safflower mayo	8	105	3	4	120	0
chopped celery and 1 lettuce leaf	0	0	0	2	2	0
on 1½ slices sourdough bread	0	13	16	64	93	0
⅔ artichoke drizzled with lemon juice	0	1	7	34	42	0
⅔ cup cooked squash with wine and Worcestershire sauce	0	3	4	23	30	0
3 vanilla wafers	0	17	0	40	57	0
Noncaloric beverage	0	0	0	0	0	0
TOTALS	8	140	58	167	373	15
Total proportions	2%	38%	15%	45%		

Dinner

½ small chicken breast	10	27	60	3	100	59
fried in 2 tsp. safflower oil	7	74	0	0	81	0
⅔ cup mashed potato	6	20	10	96	132	2
with 1½ tsp. safflower margarine	5	41	0	0	46	0
⅓ cup green beans	0	1	3	14	18	0
⅓ cup cucumber, carrots and radish	0	1	1	5	7	0
Corn on the cob (⅓ cup)	1	6	7	56	70	0
with 1½ tsp. safflower margarine	5	41	0	0	46	0

	Saturated Calories	Mono & Poly Calories	Protein Calories	Carb Calories	Total Calories	Cholesterol (mg)
²/₃ slice angel food cake (unfrosted)	0	0	11	96	107	0
Noncaloric beverage	0	0	0	0	0	0
TOTALS	34	211	92	270	607	61
Total proportions	5%	35%	15%	45%		

DAY 18

Breakfast

	Saturated Calories	Mono & Poly Calories	Protein Calories	Carb Calories	Total Calories	Cholesterol (mg)
¹/₃ cup cooked cream of wheat	0	1	6	39	46	0
with 1 tsp. safflower margarine	3	34	0	0	37	0
²/₃ cup fresh strawberries	0	0	2	29	31	0
¹/₂ slice whole wheat toast	0	6	7	31	44	0
with 1¹/₂ tsp. safflower margarine	4	43	0	0	47	0
Scant 3 Tbsp. low-fat cottage cheese	3	2	21	6	32	3
Noncaloric beverage	0	0	0	0	0	0
TOTALS	10	86	36	105	237	3
Total proportions	4%	36%	15%	45%		

Lunch

	Saturated Calories	Mono & Poly Calories	Protein Calories	Carb Calories	Total Calories	Cholesterol (mg)
¹/₂ grilled fillet of sole	0	3	38	1	42	0
with scant 1¹/₂ Tbsp. tartar sauce	0	97	0	0	97	0
on 1 sourdough roll	0	19	13	81	113	0
with 1 tomato slice	0	0	1	5	6	0
2 small roasted red potatoes	0	1	6	80	87	0
drizzled with 1¹/₂ tsp. rosemary olive oil	3	24	0	0	27	0
Noncaloric beverage	0	0	0	0	0	0
TOTALS	3	144	58	167	372	0
Total proportions	1%	39%	15%	45%		

	Saturated Calories	Mono & Poly Calories	Protein Calories	Carb Calories	Total Calories	Cholesterol (mg)
Dinner						
2 oz. lean roasted lamb	20	21	60	0	101	0
1/3 cup macaroni and cheese	32	63	21	55	171	0
1/3 cup brussels sprouts with 2 tsp. safflower margarine	0 7	2 61	6 0	20 0	28 68	0 0
1/3 cup cooked carrots with 1 tsp. safflower margarine	0 3	1 30	2 0	22 0	25 33	0 0
3/4 cup mandarin-orange sorbet	0	1	3	170	174	0
Noncaloric beverage	0	0	0	0	0	0
TOTALS	62	179	92	267	600	0
Total proportions	10%	30%	15%	45%		

DAY 19

Breakfast

	Saturated Calories	Mono & Poly Calories	Protein Calories	Carb Calories	Total Calories	Cholesterol (mg)
4 large stewed prunes topped with 1/2 tsp. safflower margarine	0 1	0 15	3 0	79 0	82 16	0 0
1/2 slice rye toast with 1 tsp. safflower margarine	0 3	4 34	5 0	26 0	35 37	0 0
1 oz. turkey sausage	13	22	27	0	62	23
Noncaloric beverage	0	0	0	0	0	0
TOTALS	17	75	35	105	232	23
Total proportions	7%	33%	15%	45%		

Lunch

	Saturated Calories	Mono & Poly Calories	Protein Calories	Carb Calories	Total Calories	Cholesterol (mg)
1.5 oz. lean grilled hamburger	24	38	41	0	103	58
1 tsp. mustard	0	1	1	2	4	0
1 generous tsp. safflower mayonnaise	0	40	0	0	40	0

	Saturated Calories	Mono & Poly Calories	Protein Calories	Carb Calories	Total Calories	Cholesterol (mg)
2 tsp. catsup	0	1	1	9	11	0
1 small dinner roll	0	13	9	54	76	0
1 small tomato	0	1	1	7	9	0
2 cucumber sticks drizzled with 1 tsp. vinaigrette	0 1	0 23	1 0	4 1	5 25	0 0
3 radishes	0	1	1	2	4	0
1 medium to small banana	0	2	3	87	92	0
Noncaloric beverage	0	0	0	0	0	0
TOTALS	25	120	58	166	369	58
Total proportions	7%	33%	15%	45%		

Dinner

	Saturated Calories	Mono & Poly Calories	Protein Calories	Carb Calories	Total Calories	Cholesterol (mg)
Generous 2 oz. turkey summer sausage fried in safflower oil (leaving residue in pan)	23 2	45 18	41 0	4 0	113 20	82 0
◆ ½ cup red cabbage	0	2	3	13	18	0
¼ cup beef broth	0	1	1	2	4	0
1 tsp. safflower margarine	3	31	0	0	34	0
1 to 2 tsp. balsamic vinegar	0	0	0	1	1	0
⅔ slice Canadian bacon, diced	5	17	31	0	53	3
⅓ tart green apple, sliced	0	1	1	28	30	0
½ tsp. brown sugar	0	0	0	6	6	0
⅔ cup garlic mashed potatoes with 1 tsp. safflower margarine	14 3	40 31	11 0	93 0	158 34	2 0
Generous ½ cup apple sauce	0	2	0	118	120	0
Noncaloric beverage	0	0	0	0	0	0
TOTALS	50	188	88	265	591	87
Total proportions	8%	32%	15%	45%		

◆   To prepare the red cabbage, shred the cabbage after removing the hard core. Soak cabbage for a few minutes in cold water. Drain and add beef broth, margarine, vinegar, Canadian bacon, brown sugar and apple. Cook on low heat until apple slices are soft and blended with the cabbage. Add salt and spices to taste.

	Saturated Calories	Mono & Poly Calories	Protein Calories	Carb Calories	Total Calories	Cholesterol (mg)

DAY 20

Breakfast

	Saturated Calories	Mono & Poly Calories	Protein Calories	Carb Calories	Total Calories	Cholesterol (mg)
1 small toasted bagel	0	11	15	70	96	0
with 2 tsp. safflower margarine	7	61	0	0	68	0
²/₃ cup low-fat milk	5	7	21	35	68	6
Noncaloric beverage	0	0	0	0	0	0
TOTALS	12	79	36	105	232	6
Total proportions	5%	35%	15%	45%		

Lunch

	Saturated Calories	Mono & Poly Calories	Protein Calories	Carb Calories	Total Calories	Cholesterol (mg)
Chicken and biscuits: 1.5 oz. stewed chicken	6	16	42	0	64	38
with 3 Tbsp. celery	0	0	0	2	2	0
3 Tbsp. carrots	0	0	1	9	10	0
3 Tbsp. onion	0	0	1	8	9	0
3 Tbsp. potato	0	0	1	16	17	0
Spices to taste (clove, allspice, bay leaf)	0	0	1	7	8	0
1½ biscuits (from mix)	0	39	11	70	120	0
with 2 tsp. safflower margarine	7	61	0	0	68	0
²/₃ oz. chocolate fudge	6	13	2	58	79	0
Noncaloric beverage	0	0	0	0	0	0
TOTALS	19	129	59	170	377	38
Total proportions	5%	35%	15%	45%		

Dinner

	Saturated Calories	Mono & Poly Calories	Protein Calories	Carb Calories	Total Calories	Cholesterol (mg)
2.2 oz. trout	7	36	58	0	101	41
dusted in 4 tsp. flour	0	0	5	36	41	0
and fried in safflower oil (leaving oil residue in pan)	7	75	0	0	82	0
4 large asparagus spears	0	1	7	14	22	0
with ½ tsp. safflower margarine and 1 tsp. lemon juice	1	17	0	0	18	0

	Saturated Calories	Mono & Poly Calories	Protein Calories	Carb Calories	Total Calories	Cholesterol (mg)
⅓ cup corn on the cob	1	6	9	56	72	0
with 1 tsp. safflower margarine	3	34	0	0	37	0
⅔ large baked potato	0	1	13	165	179	0
with 1½ tsp. safflower margarine	5	45	0	0	50	0
Noncaloric beverage	0	0	0	0	0	0
TOTALS	24	215	92	271	602	41
Total proportions	4%	36%	15%	45%		

DAY 21

Breakfast

	Saturated Calories	Mono & Poly Calories	Protein Calories	Carb Calories	Total Calories	Cholesterol (mg)
⅔ cup melon balls	0	1	3	34	38	0
1 5-in. buttermilk pancake	1	3	9	71	84	0
with 1½ tsp. safflower margarine	5	45	0	0	50	0
1 generous oz. chicken apple sausage	13	25	24	0	62	25
Noncaloric beverage	0	0	0	0	0	0
TOTALS	19	74	36	105	234	25
Total proportions	8%	32%	15%	45%		

Lunch

	Saturated Calories	Mono & Poly Calories	Protein Calories	Carb Calories	Total Calories	Cholesterol (mg)
2 oz. grilled sea bass sandwich on a sourdough roll with 1 Tbsp. tartar sauce, lettuce and tomato	2	73	53	67	195	23
⅓ cup potato salad (made with safflower mayo and oil and vinegar)	6	65	2	36	109	0
2 fresh apricots	0	1	1	31	33	0
2 small dried dates	0	0	0	33	33	0
Noncaloric beverage	0	0	0	0	0	0
TOTALS	8	139	56	167	370	23
Total proportions	2%	38%	15%	45%		

	Saturated Calories	Mono & Poly Calories	Protein Calories	Carb Calories	Total Calories	Cholesterol (mg)

Dinner

Beans and franks:						
²/₃ of 1 turkey frank	15	38	15	25	93	30
on ²/₃ hot dog bun	0	13	9	54	76	0
with 2 tsp. mustard	0	5	3	3	11	0
2 tsp. catsup	0	0	1	9	10	0
²/₃ cup baked beans	0	0	40	144	184	0
²/₃ artichoke	0	1	7	32	40	0
with 1¹/₃ Tbsp. safflower mayo with lemon to taste	14	117	1	2	134	0
1 cup mixed baby greens	0	0	0	2	2	0
with ²/₃ oz. shrimp	0	3	15	1	19	0
1¹/₂ tsp. vinaigrette	6	26	0	0	32	0
Noncaloric beverage	0	0	0	0	0	0
TOTALS	35	203	91	272	601	30
Total proportions	6%	34%	15%	45%		

DAY 22

Breakfast

¹/₂ cup cooked oatmeal with cinnamon	0	11	11	51	73	0
1¹/₂ tsp. safflower margarine	4	44	0	0	48	0
topped with 1 tsp. sliced almonds	1	12	1	2	16	0
¹/₃ cup low-fat milk	2	3	11	18	34	3
¹/₂ small grapefruit	0	1	1	30	32	0
1 thin slice Canadian bacon	5	9	13	3	30	9
Noncaloric beverage	0	0	0	0	0	0
TOTALS	12	80	37	104	233	12
Total proportions	5%	34.5%	15.5%	45%		

Lunch

Chicken burrito:						
1 oz. chicken breast	3	8	31	0	42	24
¹/₄ cup cooked rice	0	0	3	50	53	0

	Saturated Calories	Mono & Poly Calories	Protein Calories	Carb Calories	Total Calories	Cholesterol (mg)
¼ cup refried beans	2	3	15	46	66	0
1 flour tortilla	0	20	9	60	89	0
cooked in scant 1½ tsp. olive oil	5	40	0	0	45	0
⅔ cup fresh cabbage coleslaw	0	0	1	10	11	0
with 2 tsp. safflower mayo	7	59	0	0	66	0
Noncaloric beverage	0	0	0	0	0	0
TOTALS	17	130	59	166	372	24
Total proportions	5%	35%	15%	45%		

Dinner

	Saturated Calories	Mono & Poly Calories	Protein Calories	Carb Calories	Total Calories	Cholesterol (mg)
1.7 oz. pheasant (without skin)	5	11	43	0	59	0
⅔ cup wild and long-grain rice mix	28	20	14	132	194	7
2 tsp. toasted filbert nuts	0	42	8	7	57	0
3 Tbsp. burnt diced onion	0	0	1	9	10	0
sautéed in 1½ tsp. safflower oil	5	50	0	0	55	0
♦ ½ cup red cabbage	0	2	4	14	20	0
beef broth	0	1	1	2	4	0
1 to 2 tsp. balsamic vinegar	0	0	0	1	1	0
⅓ slice Canadian bacon	2	9	13	0	24	0
⅓ tart green apple	0	1	1	27	29	0
1 scant tsp. brown sugar	0	0	0	9	9	0
4 asparagus spears	0	1	6	11	18	0
topped with 1½ tsp. safflower margarine and 1 tsp. lemon juice	7	61	0	0	68	0
⅓ cup lemon sorbet	0	0	1	60	61	0
Noncaloric beverage	0	0	0	0	0	0
TOTALS	47	198	92	272	609	7
Total proportions	8%	32%	15%	45%		

♦ Prepare the red cabbage according to the instructions for this recipe on Day 19, p. 201, leaving out the margarine.

	Saturated Calories	Mono & Poly Calories	Protein Calories	Carb Calories	Total Calories	Cholesterol (mg)

DAY 23

Breakfast

	Saturated Calories	Mono & Poly Calories	Protein Calories	Carb Calories	Total Calories	Cholesterol (mg)
4 oz. fresh orange juice	0	0	3	52	55	0
½ oat bran English muffin	0	6	9	53	68	0
with 1½ tsp. safflower margarine	5	45	0	0	50	0
1 oz. turkey sausage	13	23	24	0	60	23
Noncaloric beverage	0	0	0	0	0	0
TOTALS	18	74	36	105	233	23
Total proportions	8%	32%	15%	45%		

Lunch

	Saturated Calories	Mono & Poly Calories	Protein Calories	Carb Calories	Total Calories	Cholesterol (mg)
♦ Cheese-baked tofu: ⅓-in.-thick tofu slice sprinkled with garlic tamari sauce and 1 Tbsp.	7	18	34	9	68	0
grated Gruyère or Emmentaler cheese	22	14	11	1	48	14
♦ Curried rice: ⅓ cup cooked brown rice	0	7	7	67	81	0
with onion and garlic	0	0	0	2	2	0
zucchini	0	0	0	1	1	0
shiitake mushroom	0	1	1	4	6	0
mung bean sprouts	0	0	1	4	5	0
sautéed in 2 tsp safflower oil	7	74	0	0	81	0
1 small pear	0	0	3	80	83	0
Noncaloric beverage	0	0	0	0	0	0
TOTALS	36	114	57	168	375	14
Total proportions	10%	30%	15%	45%		

♦ To prepare the tofu, preheat the oven to 350° and coat a baking tray or dish with nonstick baking spray. Set aside. Poke holes in the tofu patty with a fork and sprinkle with garlic tamari sauce. (Tamari sauce is a light and flavorful soy-based sauce that can be found in many grocery stores, especially those that stock Japanese food products.) Sprinkle the cheeses on the patty and bake until a bit crusty, or about 20 minutes.

♦ Prepare the rice according to the directions on the package. Remove from heat and keep covered. Heat oil in a skillet over medium heat. Add 2 teaspoons onion. When the onion is light golden, add half of a small clove garlic, chopped, and sauté until the onion is slightly burnt. Stir in 2 teaspoons chopped zucchini, 2 teaspoons chopped mushrooms (without the stems and soaked 15 minutes in boiling water) and 2 teaspoons mung bean sprouts. Add a pinch of curry powder, to taste. Cook, stirring frequently, for 5 minutes on medium heat. Fluff the rice with a fork and add to the skillet. Cook and stir frequently for 2 to 3 minutes. Serve.

	Saturated Calories	Mono & Poly Calories	Protein Calories	Carb Calories	Total Calories	Cholesterol (mg)
Dinner						
♦ Stir-fried vegetables and noodles: 3 Tbsp. onion	0	0	1	9	10	0
1½ tsp. safflower oil	5	48	0	0	53	0
1 small shredded red chili	0	1	3	11	15	0
⅓ shredded carrot	0	0	1	11	12	0
⅓ cup bean sprouts	0	1	2	2	5	0
Garlic, spices and 2 tsp. soy sauce	0	0	1	3	4	0
⅔ cup cooked rice noodles	0	9	9	87	105	0
1.5 oz. grilled swordfish	3	10	29	0	42	14
1 small dinner roll	0	13	7	48	68	0
2 tsp. tartar sauce	0	53	0	0	53	0
⅔ cup custard	40	47	38	79	204	74
2 vanilla wafers	0	9	0	24	33	0
Noncaloric beverage	0	0	0	0	0	0
TOTALS	48	191	91	274	604	88
Total proportions	8%	32%	15%	45%		

♦ To prepare the stir-fried vegetables, heat the oil in a skillet on medium-high heat and add the chopped onion, red chili, carrot and bean sprouts. Sauté with a dash of garlic powder or half a small minced clove garlic. Add salt and soy sauce to taste. Fry until firm to the bite (al dente). Serve over the noodles.

	Saturated Calories	Mono & Poly Calories	Protein Calories	Carb Calories	Total Calories	Cholesterol (mg)

DAY 24

Breakfast

	Saturated Calories	Mono & Poly Calories	Protein Calories	Carb Calories	Total Calories	Cholesterol (mg)
½ cup raisin bran dry cereal	0	4	10	62	76	0
with ¼ cup low-fat milk	1	2	8	14	25	2
1 small slice Canadian bacon	5	8	13	3	29	9
½ slice rye toast	0	4	5	26	35	0
with 2 tsp. safflower margarine	7	61	0	0	68	0
Noncaloric beverage	0	0	0	0	0	0
TOTALS	13	79	36	105	233	11
Total proportions	6%	34%	15%	45%		

Lunch

	Saturated Calories	Mono & Poly Calories	Protein Calories	Carb Calories	Total Calories	Cholesterol (mg)
Shrimp burrito: 1 oz. shrimp	1	5	23	1	30	43
½ cup refried beans	4	8	27	85	124	0
1 flour tortilla	0	18	9	60	87	0
cooked in 1½ tsp. olive oil	7	46	0	0	53	0
2 tortilla chips	0	1	0	13	14	0
⅔ cup cabbage coleslaw	0	0	1	10	11	0
with generous 1½ tsp. safflower mayo	6	50	0	1	57	0
Noncaloric beverage	0	0	0	0	0	0
TOTALS	18	128	60	170	376	43
Total proportions	5%	35%	15%	45%		

Dinner

	Saturated Calories	Mono & Poly Calories	Protein Calories	Carb Calories	Total Calories	Cholesterol (mg)
2 oz. roasted Cornish game hen (without the skin)	9	26	59	0	94	46
stuffed with ⅔ cup cooked wild and long-grain rice	28	21	14	132	195	7
2 tsp. filbert nuts	0	44	7	7	58	0
3 Tbsp. burnt diced onion	0	0	0	9	9	0
sautéed in 1 tsp. safflower oil	4	37	0	0	41	0
2 Tbsp. currant jelly	0	0	0	51	51	0

	Saturated Calories	Mono & Poly Calories	Protein Calories	Carb Calories	Total Calories	Cholesterol (mg)
1 artichoke dipped in 2 tsp. melted safflower margarine w/lemon to taste	0 7	2 61	11 0	50 0	63 68	0 0
1/3 cup green beans	0	1	3	13	17	0
1 vanilla wafer	0	5	0	11	16	0
Noncaloric beverage	0	0	0	0	0	0
TOTALS	48	197	94	273	612	53
Total proportions	8%	32%	15%	45%		

DAY 25

Breakfast

	Saturated Calories	Mono & Poly Calories	Protein Calories	Carb Calories	Total Calories	Cholesterol (mg)
1/3 cup cooked cream of wheat	0	1	6	39	46	0
with 1 tsp. safflower margarine	3	34	0	0	37	0
2/3 cup fresh strawberries	0	0	2	29	31	0
1/2 slice whole wheat toast	0	6	7	31	44	0
with 1 1/2 tsp. safflower margarine	4	43	0	0	47	0
Scant 3 Tbsp. low-fat cottage cheese	3	2	21	6	32	3
Noncaloric beverage	0	0	0	0	0	0
TOTALS	10	86	36	105	237	3
Total proportions	5%	35%	15%	45%		

Lunch

	Saturated Calories	Mono & Poly Calories	Protein Calories	Carb Calories	Total Calories	Cholesterol (mg)
3/4 cup spaghetti with meatballs and tomato sauce	13	48	48	106	215	11
1 cup green salad with broccoli, croutons, cucumbers, carrots, tomato slices	0	14	6	36	56	0
4 tsp. oil and vinegar dressing	0	68	0	3	71	0
2 chocolate snap cookies	0	0	1	23	24	0

	Saturated Calories	Mono & Poly Calories	Protein Calories	Carb Calories	Total Calories	Cholesterol (mg)
Noncaloric beverage	0	0	0	0	0	0
TOTALS	13	130	55	168	366	11
Total proportions	4%	36%	15%	45%		

Dinner

	Saturated Calories	Mono & Poly Calories	Protein Calories	Carb Calories	Total Calories	Cholesterol (mg)
3½ oz. corned beef with fat cut off	25	102	64	2	193	87
⅓ cup cooked cabbage	0	1	2	9	12	0
⅓ cup cooked carrots with 1 tsp. safflower margarine	0	1	3	22	26	0
	3	34	0	0	37	0
⅔ boiled potato with 1½ tsp. safflower margarine	0	1	6	72	79	0
	5	45	0	0	50	0
3 Tbsp. cooked onion	0	1	1	9	11	0
⅓ cup cooked celery	0	0	1	7	8	0
1 sliver carrot cake	0	24	13	96	133	0
with 5 tsp. glaze frosting	0	0	0	54	54	0
Noncaloric beverage	0	0	0	0	0	0
TOTALS	33	209	90	271	603	87
Total proportions	5%	35%	15%	45%		

DAY 26

Breakfast

	Saturated Calories	Mono & Poly Calories	Protein Calories	Carb Calories	Total Calories	Cholesterol (mg)
4 large stewed prunes topped with ½ tsp. safflower margarine	0	0	3	79	82	0
	1	15	0	0	16	0
½ slice rye toast with 1 tsp. safflower margarine	0	4	5	26	35	0
	3	34	0	0	37	0
1 oz. turkey sausage	13	22	27	0	62	23
Noncaloric beverage	0	0	0	0	0	0
TOTALS	17	75	35	105	232	23
Total proportions	7%	33%	15%	45%		

	Saturated Calories	Mono & Poly Calories	Protein Calories	Carb Calories	Total Calories	Cholesterol (mg)
Lunch						
Chicken salad: 1 oz. chicken breast	4	10	40	0	54	85
2 cups romaine lettuce lemon juice, wine vinegar, Worcestershire sauce, pepper and 2 generous tsp. garlic olive oil	0	0	1	6	7	0
	13	87	0	0	100	0
1/3 cup croutons	0	18	3	22	43	0
1 1/2 slices sourdough French bread	0	12	15	64	91	0
1 cup blackberries	0	1	1	74	76	0
Noncaloric beverage	0	0	0	0	0	0
TOTALS	17	128	60	166	371	85
Total proportions	5%	35%	15%	45%		
Dinner						
2/3 cup risotto (rice)	0	1	11	134	146	0
with generous 2 oz. shrimp	2	9	58	3	72	109
2 tsp. shallots	0	0	1	5	6	0
1 1/2 tsp. safflower margarine	4	41	0	0	45	0
1 1/2 tsp. olive oil	6	47	0	0	53	0
1 1/2 tsp. grated Parmesan cheese	6	3	6	1	16	3
1/2 cup chicken broth	1	3	3	3	10	1
1/3 cup zucchini squash with 1 1/2 tsp. safflower margarine	0	1	3	11	15	0
	5	41	0	0	46	0
2/3 cup four-bean salad	0	2	11	108	121	0
with 1 Tbsp. vinaigrette	0	72	0	0	72	0
Hot mint tea with 1/2 tsp. sugar	0	0	0	8	8	0
Noncaloric beverage	0	0	0	0	0	0
TOTALS	24	220	93	273	610	113
Total proportions	4%	36%	15%	45%		

	Saturated Calories	Mono & Poly Calories	Protein Calories	Carb Calories	Total Calories	Cholesterol (mg)
DAY 27						
Breakfast						
1 small toasted bagel	0	11	15	70	96	0
with 2 tsp. safflower margarine	7	61	0	0	68	0
⅔ cup low-fat milk	5	7	21	35	68	6
Noncaloric beverage	0	0	0	0	0	0
TOTALS	12	79	36	105	232	6
Total proportions	5%	35%	15%	45%		
Lunch						
⅔ grilled fillet of sole	0	2	47	1	50	0
13 french fries fried in safflower oil	27	73	9	107	216	0
½ fresh papaya	0	1	2	53	56	0
sliced onto a bed of 4 romaine lettuce leaves drizzled with 2 tsp. honey vinaigrette	7	38	0	7	52	0
Noncaloric beverage	0	0	0	0	0	0
TOTALS	34	114	58	168	374	0
Total proportions	9%	31%	15%	45%		
Dinner						
2.3 oz. lean London broil	38	51	67	0	156	47
marinated in 2 tsp. olive oil, red wine vinegar (amount absorbed)	10	69	0	0	79	0
⅔ baked potato	0	1	13	136	150	0
with 1½ tsp. safflower margarine	5	41	0	0	46	0
⅓ cup small peas	0	1	11	33	45	0
with 2 tsp. onion	0	0	0	2	2	0

	Saturated Calories	Mono & Poly Calories	Protein Calories	Carb Calories	Total Calories	Cholesterol (mg)
sautéed in a dollop of safflower margarine	2	19	0	0	21	0
²/₃ cup fresh pineapple	0	4	1	51	56	0
on top of ¼ cup pineapple or strawberry sorbet	0	0	1	49	50	0
Noncaloric beverage	0	0	0	0	0	0
TOTALS	55	186	93	271	605	47
Total proportions	9%	31%	15%	45%		

DAY 28

Breakfast

	Saturated Calories	Mono & Poly Calories	Protein Calories	Carb Calories	Total Calories	Cholesterol (mg)
²/₃ cup melon balls	0	1	3	34	38	0
1 5-in. buttermilk pancake	1	3	9	71	84	0
with 1½ tsp. safflower margarine	5	45	0	0	50	0
1 generous oz. chicken apple sausage	13	25	24	0	62	25
Noncaloric beverage	0	0	0	0	0	0
TOTALS	19	74	36	105	234	25
Total proportions	8%	32%	15%	45%		

Lunch

	Saturated Calories	Mono & Poly Calories	Protein Calories	Carb Calories	Total Calories	Cholesterol (mg)
Generous ²/₃ cup black bean chili	1	5	46	130	182	0
cooked with chicken broth and 3 Tbsp. onion	0	0	0	8	8	0
3 Tbsp. bell pepper	0	0	0	3	3	0
⅓ cup fresh tomato	0	0	1	7	8	0
sautéed in 1 generous tsp. safflower oil,	10	120	0	0	130	0
1 Tbsp. tomato paste	0	1	3	12	16	0
and a dash each of oregano, cumin, paprika, coriander, ½ bay leaf, salt, pepper, ½ tsp. chili powder and 1 tsp. red wine vinegar	0	0	1	6	7	0
topped with 1 Tbsp. Parmesan cheese	8	4	8	1	21	4

	Saturated Calories	Mono & Poly Calories	Protein Calories	Carb Calories	Total Calories	Cholesterol (mg)
Noncaloric beverage	0	0	0	0	0	0
TOTALS	19	130	59	167	375	4
Total proportions	5%	35%	15%	45%		

To prepare, see instructions in the 1,800 calorie diet for Day 28 Lunch, p. 260; substitute the above proportions.

Dinner

	Saturated Calories	Mono & Poly Calories	Protein Calories	Carb Calories	Total Calories	Cholesterol (mg)
2 oz. halibut steak	3	12	59	0	74	23
baked crusty with equal mixture cornmeal and flour	0	0	1	7	8	0
and 1 tsp. melted safflower margarine	3	30	0	0	33	0
²/₃ cup cooked rice	0	1	10	133	144	0
with 1¹/₂ Tbsp. pineapple	0	0	0	7	7	0
2 tsp. toasted pine nuts	8	45	4	7	64	0
¹/₃ cup green peas	0	1	10	33	44	0
with 1 tsp. safflower margarine	3	30	0	0	33	0
²/₃ small sweet potato	0	0	3	46	49	0
with 1¹/₂ tsp. safflower margarine	4	41	0	0	45	0
1 small dinner roll	0	12	6	37	55	0
with 1¹/₂ tsp. safflower margarine	4	41	0	0	45	0
Noncaloric beverage	0	0	0	0	0	0
TOTALS	25	213	93	270	601	23
Total proportions	4%	36%	15%	45%		

DAY 29

Breakfast

	Saturated Calories	Mono & Poly Calories	Protein Calories	Carb Calories	Total Calories	Cholesterol (mg)
¹/₂ cup cooked oatmeal with cinnamon	0	11	11	51	73	0
1¹/₂ tsp. safflower margarine	4	44	0	0	48	0
topped with 1 tsp. sliced almonds	1	12	1	2	16	0

	Saturated Calories	Mono & Poly Calories	Protein Calories	Carb Calories	Total Calories	Cholesterol (mg)
1/3 cup low-fat milk	2	3	11	18	34	3
1/2 small grapefruit	0	1	1	30	32	0
1 slice Canadian bacon	5	9	13	3	30	9
Noncaloric beverage	0	0	0	0	0	0
TOTALS	12	80	37	104	233	12
Total proportions	5%	34.5%	15.5%	45%		

Lunch

	Saturated Calories	Mono & Poly Calories	Protein Calories	Carb Calories	Total Calories	Cholesterol (mg)
Crab salad: 2 oz. crab	0	2	42	0	44	23
marinated in vinaigrette of						
2 scant tsp. Dijon mustard	0	3	1	1	5	0
2 tsp. minced shallots	0	0	0	4	4	0
2 tsp. white wine vinegar	0	0	0	1	1	0
2 tsp. olive oil	8	70	0	0	78	0
set on 4 prebaked potato						
slices	1	2	12	157	172	0
sautéed in olive oil (leave						
residue in pan)	7	55	0	0	62	0
on bed of 1/3 cup fresh						
spinach	0	0	1	3	4	0
Noncaloric beverage	0	0	0	0	0	0
TOTALS	16	132	56	166	370	23
Total proportions	4%	36%	15%	45%		

Dinner

	Saturated Calories	Mono & Poly Calories	Protein Calories	Carb Calories	Total Calories	Cholesterol (mg)
Orange-baked chicken:						
1 small half breast of						
chicken (without the skin)	4	12	65	0	81	44
baked with 2 tsp. orange						
juice concentrate	0	0	2	33	35	0
2 tsp. safflower margarine						
and spices	7	60	0	0	67	0
1/3 cup stir-fried mixed						
vegetables	0	1	6	20	27	0
in 1 tsp. peanut oil	5	34	0	0	39	0
1/2 cup white rice	0	1	8	100	109	0
and 1/2 tsp. safflower						
margarine cooked in						
chicken broth	1	15	0	0	16	0

	Saturated Calories	Mono & Poly Calories	Protein Calories	Carb Calories	Total Calories	Cholesterol (mg)
2 tsp. burnt onion sautéed in ½ tsp. safflower	0	0	0	4	4	0
margarine	1	15	0	0	16	0
2 oz. date nut cake	0	90	13	114	217	46
Noncaloric beverage	0	0	0	0	0	0
TOTALS	18	228	94	271	611	90
Total proportions	3%	37%	15%	45%		

DAY 30

Breakfast

	Saturated Calories	Mono & Poly Calories	Protein Calories	Carb Calories	Total Calories	Cholesterol (mg)
4 oz. fresh orange juice	0	0	3	52	55	0
½ oat bran English muffin with 1½ generous tsp.	0	6	9	53	68	0
safflower margarine	5	45	0	0	50	0
1 oz. turkey sausage	13	23	24	0	60	23
Noncaloric beverage	0	0	0	0	0	0
TOTALS	18	74	36	105	233	23
Total proportions	8%	32%	15%	45%		

Lunch

	Saturated Calories	Mono & Poly Calories	Protein Calories	Carb Calories	Total Calories	Cholesterol (mg)
1.7 oz turkey breast sandwich	4	7	38	2	51	17
¼ small avocado	7	46	3	8	64	0
2 tsp. safflower mayo	6	59	0	1	66	0
on rye roll	0	17	18	106	141	0
⅔ apple	0	0	0	52	52	0
Noncaloric beverage	0	0	0	0	0	0
TOTALS	17	129	59	169	374	17
Total proportions	5%	35%	15%	45%		

Dinner

	Saturated Calories	Mono & Poly Calories	Protein Calories	Carb Calories	Total Calories	Cholesterol (mg)
2.3 oz. broiled lobster dipped in 5 tsp. safflower margarine and lemon	0	3	55	3	61	48
juice	18	152	0	0	170	0
4 chilled asparagus spears topped with 1½ tsp. yogurt	0	1	6	11	18	0
dressing	3	2	3	3	11	3
2 quick-boiled tomato halves topped with 2 tsp. grated	0	3	4	21	28	0
Parmesan cheese	6	3	5	1	15	3
1½ small sourdough rolls	0	25	12	75	112	0
⅔ cup orange sorbet	14	8	6	157	185	9
Noncaloric beverage	0	0	0	0	0	0
TOTALS	41	197	91	271	600	63
Total proportions	7%	33%	15%	45%		

SIXTEEN

MENU PLANS FOR

THE 1,800 CALORIE DIET

DAY 1

Breakfast

	Saturated Calories	Mono & Poly Calories	Protein Calories	Carb Calories	Total Calories	Cholesterol (mg)
½ cup cooked oatmeal with cinnamon	0	11	11	51	73	0
topped with 2 tsp. sliced almonds	1	24	1	4	30	0
⅓ cup low-fat milk	2	3	11	18	34	3
½ grapefruit	0	1	1	34	36	0
1 slice whole wheat toast	0	9	10	45	64	0
with 2 tsp. safflower margarine	7	61	0	0	68	0
1 slice Canadian bacon	7	12	19	4	42	13
Noncaloric beverage	0	0	0	0	0	0
TOTALS	17	121	53	156	347	16
Total proportions	5%	35%	15%	45%		

Note: Each menu yields 1 serving.

	Saturated Calories	Mono & Poly Calories	Protein Calories	Carb Calories	Total Calories	Cholesterol (mg)

Lunch

	Saturated Calories	Mono & Poly Calories	Protein Calories	Carb Calories	Total Calories	Cholesterol (mg)
Peanut butter sandwich special: 2 Tbsp. peanut butter	40	106	26	18	190	0
1 Tbsp. honey	0	0	0	64	64	0
1/3 cup green seedless grapes cut in halves	0	1	0	18	19	0
between 2 slices buttermilk white toast	0	12	24	104	140	0
Green salad with 1 cup lettuce	0	0	1	7	8	0
4 tomato wedges	0	0	0	4	4	0
cucumber slices	0	0	0	2	2	0
3 Tbsp. small cooked shrimp	1	5	34	1	41	65
2 tsp. vinaigrette	0	47	0	1	48	0
1 Nabisco gingersnap	1	3	1	25	30	0
Noncaloric beverage	0	0	0	0	0	0
TOTALS	42	174	86	244	546	65
Total proportions	8%	32%	15%	45%		

Dinner

	Saturated Calories	Mono & Poly Calories	Protein Calories	Carb Calories	Total Calories	Cholesterol (mg)
2.5 oz. roasted turkey breast with no skin	6	16	90	0	112	49
1/4 cup cranberry sauce	0	1	5	100	106	0
3/4 cup mashed potatoes	8	29	6	117	160	2
with 2 tsp. safflower margarine	7	61	0	0	68	0
1/4 baked yam with 2 tsp. safflower margarine	7	64	2	34	107	3
1/2 cup fresh peas	0	3	14	46	63	0
with 1 heaping tsp. safflower margarine	4	39	0	0	43	0
1/8 of a pumpkin pie	41	75	18	112	246	0
Noncaloric beverage	0	0	0	0	0	0
TOTALS	73	288	135	409	905	54
Total proportions	8%	32%	15%	45%		

	Saturated Calories	Mono & Poly Calories	Protein Calories	Carb Calories	Total Calories	Cholesterol (mg)

DAY 2

Breakfast

	Saturated Calories	Mono & Poly Calories	Protein Calories	Carb Calories	Total Calories	Cholesterol (mg)
4 oz. fresh orange juice	0	0	3	52	55	0
1 oat bran English muffin	0	11	19	98	128	0
with 2 generous tsp. safflower margarine	8	66	0	0	74	3
1.5 oz. turkey sausage	20	33	37	0	90	34
Noncaloric beverage	0	0	0	0	0	0
TOTALS	28	110	59	150	347	37
Total proportions	8%	32%	17%	43%		

Lunch

	Saturated Calories	Mono & Poly Calories	Protein Calories	Carb Calories	Total Calories	Cholesterol (mg)
Turkey Waldorf sandwich: 3 oz. sliced turkey	10	11	69	2	92	30
with 2 Tbsp. safflower mayo	15	170	5	8	198	0
chopped celery, walnuts, apple and lemon juice	1	8	1	1	11	0
on 2 slices thin wheat toast	0	10	10	85	105	0
1 cup grapes	0	0	1	60	61	0
2 dried dates	0	0	1	49	50	0
2 Nabisco gingersnaps	0	0	1	49	50	0
Noncaloric beverage	0	0	0	0	0	0
TOTALS	26	199	88	254	567	30
Total proportions	5%	35%	15%	45%		

Dinner

	Saturated Calories	Mono & Poly Calories	Protein Calories	Carb Calories	Total Calories	Cholesterol (mg)
Chick-peas, sausage and spinach: 1 cup cooked chick-peas	5	53	86	270	414	0
with 1/3 cup onion and 1/2 tsp. cinnamon	0	1	2	14	17	0
1 medium fresh or canned tomato	0	1	4	21	26	0
1 cup fresh spinach (packed)	0	0	6	8	14	0
2 Tbsp. golden raisins	0	0	2	57	59	0

	Saturated Calories	Mono & Poly Calories	Protein Calories	Carb Calories	Total Calories	Cholesterol (mg)
sautéed in 1½ Tbsp. olive oil with spices to taste	24	156	0	0	180	0
1 small link Italian sausage	42	72	25	1	140	34
1 piece cornbread, about 1 by 2 in. (from mix)	0	13	14	40	67	0
Noncaloric beverage	0	0	0	0	0	0
TOTALS	71	296	139	411	917	34
Total proportions	8%	32%	15%	45%		

DAY 3

Breakfast

	Saturated Calories	Mono & Poly Calories	Protein Calories	Carb Calories	Total Calories	Cholesterol (mg)
¾ cup raisin bran dry cereal	0	6	16	93	115	0
with ⅓ cup low-fat milk	2	3	11	18	34	3
1 slice Canadian bacon	7	12	19	4	42	13
1 slice rye toast	0	8	9	49	66	0
with 1 Tbsp. safflower margarine	11	91	0	0	102	0
Noncaloric beverage	0	0	0	0	0	0
TOTALS	20	120	55	164	359	16
Total proportions	6%	34%	15%	45%		

Lunch

	Saturated Calories	Mono & Poly Calories	Protein Calories	Carb Calories	Total Calories	Cholesterol (mg)
Ham and coleslaw sandwich: 3 oz. sliced cured ham	11	35	63	0	109	33
layered with ¾ cup shredded cabbage	0	0	2	11	13	0
mixed with 5 Tbsp. safflower mayo	12	141	4	8	165	0
on 2 slices pumpernickel bread	0	14	20	124	158	0
1⅓ cups fresh pineapple	0	8	2	102	112	0
Noncaloric beverage	0	0	0	0	0	0
TOTALS	23	198	91	245	557	33
Total proportions	4%	36%	16%	44%		

	Saturated Calories	Mono & Poly Calories	Protein Calories	Carb Calories	Total Calories	Cholesterol (mg)
Dinner						
Tuna kebabs: 3 oz. fresh broiled tuna	10	28	79	0	117	32
with 4 cherry tomatoes	0	1	1	10	12	0
and ½ cup eggplant	0	0	1	10	11	0
drizzled with 1 Tbsp. garlic olive oil with vinegar and oregano	13	106	0	0	119	0
over 1 cup cooked rice	0	2	16	205	223	0
2 cups lettuce and spinach salad with 1 slice Canadian bacon, chopped	6	12	28	9	55	13
and 1 Tbsp. vinaigrette	10	72	1	2	85	0
1 large sourdough roll	0	9	10	112	131	0
½ cup summer squash	0	0	1	12	13	0
stir-fried in 2 generous tsp. olive oil	10	80	0	0	90	0
1 cup fresh strawberries	0	2	1	42	45	0
Noncaloric beverage	0	0	0	0	0	0
TOTALS	49	312	138	402	901	45
Total proportions	5%	35%	15%	45%		

DAY 4

Breakfast

	Saturated Calories	Mono & Poly Calories	Protein Calories	Carb Calories	Total Calories	Cholesterol (mg)
½ cup cooked cream of wheat	0	2	8	57	67	0
with 1½ tsp. safflower margarine	5	45	0	0	50	0
1 cup fresh strawberries	0	1	2	42	45	0
1 slice whole wheat toast	0	9	10	45	64	0
with 2 tsp. safflower margarine	7	61	0	0	68	0
¼ cup low-fat cottage cheese	4	3	31	8	46	5
Noncaloric beverage	0	0	0	0	0	0
TOTALS	16	121	51	152	340	5
Total proportions	5%	35%	15%	45%		

	Saturated Calories	Mono & Poly Calories	Protein Calories	Carb Calories	Total Calories	Cholesterol (mg)
Lunch						
Chicken Dijon salad sandwich: 2 oz. white-meat chicken	4	10	74	10	98	48
2 Tbsp. safflower mayo	15	170	5	8	198	0
½ tsp. Dijon mustard	0	0	0	2	2	0
green onions, dill	0	0	0	2	2	0
1 lettuce leaf	0	0	0	2	2	0
2 slices tomato	0	0	0	7	7	0
on 2 slices French bread	0	21	17	124	162	0
1 fresh pear	0	1	1	96	98	0
Noncaloric beverage	0	0	0	0	0	0
TOTALS	19	202	97	251	569	48
Total proportions	3%	37%	17%	44%		

Dinner						
4½ oz. corned beef with fat cut off	38	152	95	3	288	130
½ cup cooked cabbage	0	1	3	14	18	0
½ cup cooked carrots with 1 tsp. safflower margarine	0	1	4	33	38	0
	3	34	0	0	37	0
1 boiled potato with 1 Tbsp. safflower margarine	0	1	9	108	118	0
	11	91	0	0	102	0
¼ cup cooked onion	0	1	2	12	15	0
½ cup cooked celery	0	0	2	10	12	0
1 slice carrot cake with 2½ tsp. glaze frosting	0	36	20	144	200	0
	0	0	0	80	80	0
Noncaloric beverage	0	0	0	0	0	0
TOTALS	52	317	135	404	908	130
Total proportions	5%	35%	15%	45%		

	Saturated Calories	Mono & Poly Calories	Protein Calories	Carb Calories	Total Calories	Cholesterol (mg)

DAY 5

Breakfast

	Saturated Calories	Mono & Poly Calories	Protein Calories	Carb Calories	Total Calories	Cholesterol (mg)
1 oz. shredded wheat dry cereal	0	5	9	88	102	0
with 1/3 cup low-fat milk	2	3	11	18	34	3
3 stewed prunes	0	0	1	53	54	0
topped with 2 tsp. safflower margarine	7	61	0	0	68	0
Scant 1.5 oz. turkey sausage	20	33	31	0	84	34
cooked in a dab of safflower margarine	1	5	0	0	6	0
Noncaloric beverage	0	0	0	0	0	0
TOTALS	30	107	52	159	348	37
Total proportions	9%	31%	15%	45%		

Lunch

	Saturated Calories	Mono & Poly Calories	Protein Calories	Carb Calories	Total Calories	Cholesterol (mg)
Vegetable stew:						
1/2 cup sweet potato	0	0	4	55	59	0
sautéed with 1 Tbsp. onion	0	0	0	3	3	0
1/2 cup zucchini	0	1	2	12	15	0
1/3 cup red bell pepper	0	1	1	8	10	0
1/2 cup baby lima beans	1	2	29	79	111	0
1/2 cup green beans	0	2	5	20	27	0
3/4 tsp. curry powder, dash saffron, salt, and other spices to taste and 1 Tbsp. olive oil	14	105	0	0	119	0
1/2 tsp. sesame oil and vegetable stock	2	18	0	0	20	0
1 slice toasted French bread	0	8	12	60	80	0
brushed with 1 tsp. garlic olive oil	5	35	0	0	40	0
with 1/4 cup diced tomato	0	0	2	11	13	0
marinated in 1 tsp. balsamic vinaigrette	1	11	0	0	12	0
1 oz. fresh grilled tuna	2	10	28	0	40	11
Noncaloric beverage	0	0	0	0	0	0
TOTALS	25	193	83	248	549	11
Total proportions	5%	35%	15%	45%		

	Saturated Calories	Mono & Poly Calories	Protein Calories	Carb Calories	Total Calories	Cholesterol (mg)

Dinner

	Saturated Calories	Mono & Poly Calories	Protein Calories	Carb Calories	Total Calories	Cholesterol (mg)
1 cup gazpacho soup	2	18	2	35	57	0
1 chicken enchilada with 1¾ oz. white meat in red sauce and salsa	15	150	72	67	304	42
1 cup cooked rice	0	2	16	205	223	0
½ cup refried beans	4	9	32	88	133	0
with 2 tsp. olive oil	9	71	0	0	80	0
1 cup green salad with 1 Tbsp. bacon bits	0	11	14	12	37	0
and 1 Tbsp. oil and vinegar dressing	13	59	0	1	73	0
Noncaloric beverage	0	0	0	0	0	0
TOTALS	43	320	136	408	907	42
Total proportions	5%	35%	15%	45%		

DAY 6

Breakfast

	Saturated Calories	Mono & Poly Calories	Protein Calories	Carb Calories	Total Calories	Cholesterol (mg)
1 large toasted bagel	0	16	24	122	162	0
with 2½ tsp. safflower margarine	9	78	0	0	87	0
and 4 tsp. light cream cheese	12	12	10	5	39	10
mixed with 1 heaping Tbsp. low-fat cottage cheese	8	7	14	3	32	1
½ cup apple slices	0	0	0	30	30	0
Noncaloric beverage	0	0	0	0	0	0
TOTALS	29	113	48	160	350	11
Total proportions	8%	32%	14%	46%		

Lunch

	Saturated Calories	Mono & Poly Calories	Protein Calories	Carb Calories	Total Calories	Cholesterol (mg)
♦ Greek tofu spinach pie: whole wheat crust	0	5	14	85	104	0
safflower oil	11	136	0	0	147	0
garlic, salt, lemon juice, minced onion	0	0	1	8	9	0

	Saturated Calories	Mono & Poly Calories	Protein Calories	Carb Calories	Total Calories	Cholesterol (mg)
Greek olives	0	12	0	9	21	0
firm tofu	10	27	50	14	101	0
fresh cooked spinach	0	1	2	4	7	0
1 sourdough roll	0	8	12	76	96	0
2 ladyfinger cookies	4	10	6	58	78	0
Noncaloric beverage	0	0	0	0	0	0
TOTALS	25	199	85	254	563	0
Total proportions	4%	36%	15%	45%		

♦ The ingredients listed above represent one-sixth of the pie, or one serving. The recipe below makes a whole pie.

Preheat oven to 350°. Use a 9-inch whole wheat piecrust, made with canola or safflower oil, which you can make or purchase.

To prepare the filling: in a large bowl mix 4 scant tablespoons safflower oil, 1 teaspoon minced garlic or garlic powder, 2 teaspoons salt, 2 tablespoons fresh lemon juice, and 12 chopped Greek olives. Add 1 pound very firm and crumbled tofu. Set it aside to marinate.

Sauté 2 tablespoons olive oil and 1 cup minced onion until the onion is slightly burnt. Add 3 cups fresh chopped spinach. Sauté 2½ minutes. Add to the tofu mixture. Transfer into the prebaked piecrust and spread out evenly, firming the mixture level. Bake for 30 minutes at 350°.

Dinner

	Saturated Calories	Mono & Poly Calories	Protein Calories	Carb Calories	Total Calories	Cholesterol (mg)
Lamb fondue: 2.25 oz. lamb with fat trimmed	23	17	76	0	116	0
½ Tbsp. safflower oil (residue from cooking lamb)	5	55	0	0	60	0
1 cup rice pilaf	0	2	16	198	216	0
with ¼ cup onion	0	0	1	12	13	0
2 tsp. safflower margarine	7	61	0	0	68	0
Dipping sauces for lamb: 2 Tbsp. yogurt chutney	10	6	8	5	29	8
2 Tbsp. dill chutney mixed with 1 Tbsp. safflower oil and Dijon mustard to taste	10	116	3	4	133	0
½ cup brussels sprouts	1	3	8	28	40	0

	Saturated Calories	Mono & Poly Calories	Protein Calories	Carb Calories	Total Calories	Cholesterol (mg)
1 artichoke dipped in lemon juice	0	2	11	50	63	0
1 thin slice carrot cake, unfrosted	13	32	13	109	167	0
Noncaloric beverage	0	0	0	0	0	0
TOTALS	69	294	136	406	905	8
Total proportions	7%	33%	15%	45%		

DAY 7

Breakfast

	Saturated Calories	Mono & Poly Calories	Protein Calories	Carb Calories	Total Calories	Cholesterol (mg)
1 cup melon balls	0	1	4	50	55	0
2 4-in. buttermilk pancakes with 2 tsp. safflower margarine	3	4	13	106	126	0
	7	61	0	0	68	0
2 oz. chicken apple sausage	20	38	34	0	92	38
Noncaloric beverage	0	0	0	0	0	0
TOTALS	30	104	51	156	341	38
Total proportions	9%	31%	15%	45%		

Lunch

	Saturated Calories	Mono & Poly Calories	Protein Calories	Carb Calories	Total Calories	Cholesterol (mg)
Grilled chicken breast sandwich: 1 small breast	4	20	65	0	89	49
with 2 Tbsp. cranberry-orange relish	0	0	0	66	66	0
on onion roll	0	20	25	145	190	0
Green salad with 1 cup lettuce	0	0	0	10	10	0
10 Greek olives	3	55	0	7	65	0
cucumber slices	0	0	0	2	2	0
3 tomato wedges	0	0	0	4	4	0
and 5 tsp. raspberry vinaigrette	0	120	0	8	128	0
Noncaloric beverage	0	0	0	0	0	0
TOTALS	7	215	90	242	554	49
Total proportions	1%	39%	16%	44%		

	Saturated Calories	Mono & Poly Calories	Protein Calories	Carb Calories	Total Calories	Cholesterol (mg)

Dinner

♦ Tuna sauce spaghetti:						
½ cup canned tomatoes with juice	0	2	3	33	38	0
garlic, 1 Tbsp. parsley	0	0	0	1	1	0
1 Tbsp. olive oil	19	127	0	0	146	0
3 oz. fresh or canned tuna with spices to taste	10	28	79	0	117	32
on 3 oz. spaghetti	0	15	43	253	311	0
1 slice garlic bread with 1 Tbsp. safflower margarine	0	9	12	48	69	0
	11	91	0	0	102	0
1 cup mixed baby greens with 2 tsp. vinaigrette	0	0	0	2	2	0
	9	39	0	1	49	0
⅔ cup black grapes	1	3	2	70	76	0
Noncaloric beverage	0	0	0	0	0	0
TOTALS	50	314	139	408	911	32
Total proportions	5%	35%	15%	45%		

♦ For spaghetti, amounts listed above are for a single serving.
Increase ingredients proportionately by the number of 1,800 calorie servings you wish to prepare.

DAY 8

Breakfast

½ cup cooked oatmeal with cinnamon	0	11	11	51	73	0
topped with 2 tsp. sliced almonds	1	24	1	4	30	0
⅓ cup lowfat milk	2	3	11	18	34	3
½ grapefruit	0	1	1	34	36	0
1 slice whole wheat toast with 2 tsp. safflower margarine	0	9	10	45	64	0
	7	61	0	0	68	0
1 slice Canadian bacon	7	12	19	4	42	13
Noncaloric beverage	0	0	0	0	0	0
TOTALS	17	121	53	156	347	16
Total proportions	5%	35%	15%	45%		

	Saturated Calories	Mono & Poly Calories	Protein Calories	Carb Calories	Total Calories	Cholesterol (mg)
Lunch						
Lamb burger: 2 oz. grilled lean lamb patty	18	16	64	0	98	0
with 1 tsp. mustard	0	1	1	2	4	0
and 1 Tbsp. catsup	0	1	1	14	16	0
on a hamburger roll	0	20	10	82	112	0
3 cucumber slices	0	0	1	6	7	0
1 medium tomato	0	3	3	22	28	0
drizzled with 4 tsp. vinaigrette	0	98	0	2	100	0
10 Greek olives	5	55	1	4	65	0
5 radishes	0	1	1	3	5	0
1 medium to large banana	1	3	5	115	124	0
Noncaloric beverage	0	0	0	0	0	0
TOTALS	24	198	87	250	559	0
Total proportions	4%	36%	15%	45%		
Dinner						
1 cup lentil soup topped with 1 Tbsp. yogurt	9	20	39	94	162	7
3.5 oz. lean ham	13	34	73	0	120	36
1 baked potato	0	1	16	203	220	0
with 1 Tbsp. safflower margarine	11	91	0	0	102	0
2 cups green salad with red onions, 1/2 oz. feta cheese, 4 tomato slices drizzled with 2 Tbsp. oil and vinegar dressing	44	126	8	10	188	12
1 minted fresh pear poached in grapefruit juice	0	6	2	100	108	0
Noncaloric beverage	0	0	0	0	0	0
TOTALS	77	278	138	407	900	55
Total proportions	9%	31%	15%	45%		

	Saturated Calories	Mono & Poly Calories	Protein Calories	Carb Calories	Total Calories	Cholesterol (mg)

DAY 9

Breakfast

	Saturated Calories	Mono & Poly Calories	Protein Calories	Carb Calories	Total Calories	Cholesterol (mg)
4 oz. fresh orange juice	0	0	3	52	55	0
1 oat bran English muffin	0	11	19	98	128	0
with 2 generous tsp. safflower margarine	8	66	0	0	74	3
1.5 oz. turkey sausage	20	33	37	0	90	34
Noncaloric beverage	0	0	0	0	0	0
TOTALS	28	110	59	150	347	37
Total proportions	8%	32%	17%	43%		

Lunch

	Saturated Calories	Mono & Poly Calories	Protein Calories	Carb Calories	Total Calories	Cholesterol (mg)
Tuna salad pita pocket: 2 oz. fresh or canned light tuna	6	19	53	0	78	21
1 pita pocket	0	8	16	82	106	0
2 Tbsp. safflower mayo	15	170	5	8	198	0
chopped onion and celery	0	0	0	4	4	0
alfalfa sprouts	0	0	0	1	1	0
1 slice tomato	0	0	1	5	6	0
cucumber slices	0	0	0	1	1	0
½ cup mandarin oranges	0	5	5	27	37	0
mixed with 2 Tbsp. vanilla yogurt	0	0	1	82	83	0
3 Nabisco chocolate snap cookies	0	0	2	34	36	0
Noncaloric beverage	0	0	0	0	0	0
TOTALS	21	202	83	244	550	21
Total proportions	4%	36%	15%	45%		

Dinner

	Saturated Calories	Mono & Poly Calories	Protein Calories	Carb Calories	Total Calories	Cholesterol (mg)
2.5 oz. lean rib roast beef with fat trimmed	37	52	78	0	167	81
1 large baked potato	1	2	25	271	299	0
with 2½ tsp. safflower margarine	9	77	0	0	86	0
2 cup mixed greens	0	2	6	16	24	0

	Saturated Calories	Mono & Poly Calories	Protein Calories	Carb Calories	Total Calories	Cholesterol (mg)
1 Tbsp. grated carrot	0	0	0	7	7	0
½ tomato cut in wedges	0	1	2	10	13	0
1 Tbsp. Italian dressing	9	55	0	6	70	0
2 pieces garlic bread made with 1 Tbsp.	0	18	24	100	142	0
safflower margarine	11	91	0	0	102	0
Noncaloric beverage	0	0	0	0	0	0
TOTALS	67	298	135	410	910	81
Total proportions	7%	33%	15%	45%		

DAY 10

Breakfast

	Saturated Calories	Mono & Poly Calories	Protein Calories	Carb Calories	Total Calories	Cholesterol (mg)
¾ cup raisin bran dry cereal	0	6	16	93	115	0
with ⅓ cup low-fat milk	2	3	11	18	34	3
1 slice Canadian bacon	7	12	19	4	42	13
1 slice rye toast with 1 Tbsp. safflower	0	8	9	49	66	0
margarine	11	91	0	0	102	0
Noncaloric beverage	0	0	0	0	0	0
TOTALS	20	120	55	164	359	16
Total proportions	6%	34%	15%	45%		

Lunch

	Saturated Calories	Mono & Poly Calories	Protein Calories	Carb Calories	Total Calories	Cholesterol (mg)
1 chicken or turkey hot dog	23	49	23	3	98	39
1 bun	0	19	14	81	114	0
1 Tbsp. mustard	0	8	4	4	16	0
1 Tbsp. catsup	0	1	1	20	22	0
⅓ cup potato salad made with safflower mayo and oil and vinegar	5	63	2	45	115	0
1 cup New England clam chowder	25	30	38	60	153	22
2 Nabisco chocolate snap cookies	0	0	2	34	36	0
Noncaloric beverage	0	0	0	0	0	0
TOTALS	53	170	84	247	554	61
Total proportions	9%	31%	15%	45%		

	Saturated Calories	Mono & Poly Calories	Protein Calories	Carb Calories	Total Calories	Cholesterol (mg)
Dinner						
3.8 oz. fresh salmon	8	48	82	0	138	59
broiled with 2 tsp. olive oil	10	68	0	0	78	0
1 small baked potato	0	0	16	149	165	0
with 1 Tbsp. safflower margarine	11	91	0	0	102	0
1 cup green beans	0	0	8	31	39	0
and 1 Tbsp. olive oil mixed with lemon juice to taste	11	68	0	0	79	0
1 sourdough roll	0	8	12	80	100	0
with 1 tsp. safflower margarine	3	34	0	0	37	0
1 slice angel food cake	0	0	17	144	161	0
Noncaloric beverage	0	0	0	0	0	0
TOTALS	43	317	135	404	899	59
Total proportions	5%	35%	15%	45%		

DAY 11

Breakfast

	Saturated Calories	Mono & Poly Calories	Protein Calories	Carb Calories	Total Calories	Cholesterol (mg)
½ cup cooked cream of wheat	0	2	8	57	67	0
with 1½ tsp. safflower margarine	5	45	0	0	50	0
1 cup fresh strawberries	0	1	2	42	45	0
1 slice whole wheat toast	0	9	10	45	64	0
with 2 tsp. safflower margarine	7	61	0	0	68	0
¼ cup low-fat cottage cheese	4	3	31	8	46	5
Noncaloric beverage	0	0	0	0	0	0
TOTALS	16	121	51	152	340	5
Total proportions	5%	35%	15%	45%		

	Saturated Calories	Mono & Poly Calories	Protein Calories	Carb Calories	Total Calories	Cholesterol (mg)
Lunch						
♦ Vegetable tofu burgers: 1 generous Tbsp. sesame oil	18	122	0	0	140	0
burnt onion, carrot, garlic and water chestnuts	0	1	2	14	17	0
½ cup chopped fresh spinach	0	1	2	4	7	0
⅓ cup firm (not silken) tofu	10	27	50	14	101	0
2 tsp. toasted sesame seeds	3	23	6	2	34	0
on focaccia (flat bread) or thin-sliced toasted sourdough bread	0	17	20	87	124	0
Fruit salad with 1 medium fresh peach	0	0	0	37	37	0
½ fresh papaya	0	0	2	60	62	0
and ⅓ banana	0	0	1	33	34	0
Noncaloric beverage	0	0	0	0	0	0
TOTALS	31	191	83	251	556	0
Total proportions	5%	35%	15%	45%		

♦ This recipe is for 1 patty. Increase the proportions according to how many patties you wish to prepare. Preheat oven to 350°. Coat a baking tray with nonstick cooking spray and set aside.

Sauté 1 tablespoon minced onion in sesame oil until slightly burnt. Add 1 tablespoon peeled and grated carrot and sauté for 4 to 5 minutes. Add ⅛ teaspoon salt, ⅛ teaspoon garlic powder, 1 tablespoon chopped water chestnuts and the spinach. Crumble the tofu in a food processor. Mix the crumbled tofu into the other ingredients. Add the toasted sesame seeds. Form mixture into a patty. Bake at 350° on the oiled tray for 25 minutes or until golden brown. Serve on a roll or focaccia (flat bread).

Dinner

	Saturated Calories	Mono & Poly Calories	Protein Calories	Carb Calories	Total Calories	Cholesterol (mg)
⅓ to ½ cup chicken, cubed and stir-fried in	6	18	42	8	74	27
2 tsp. canola or sesame oil	6	70	0	0	76	0
and rolled in 1 Tbsp. sesame seeds	5	34	8	3	50	0

	Saturated Calories	Mono & Poly Calories	Protein Calories	Carb Calories	Total Calories	Cholesterol (mg)
♦ Udon soup:						
1 to 3 shiitake mushrooms	0	1	3	31	35	0
1/3 cup green cabbage	0	3	6	17	26	0
1/2 cup spinach or collard greens	0	2	6	20	28	0
1/4 cup firm tofu, cubed	7	43	40	11	101	0
1 cup cooked Udon noodles (thick white noodles)	0	22	26	150	198	50
Pinch of hot pepper and 1 1/2 tsp. tahini	4	63	5	6	78	0
1/2 tsp. miso	0	0	1	4	5	0
1/2 tsp. tamari sauce	0	0	0	1	1	0
2 tsp. sesame oil with garlic to taste	6	70	0	0	76	0
1/8 tsp. onion powder	0	0	0	0	0	0
3/4 cup strawberry sorbet	0	1	2	152	155	0
Noncaloric beverage	0	0	0	0	0	0
TOTALS	34	327	139	403	903	77
Total proportions	4%	36%	15%	45%		

♦ Place the shiitake mushroom pieces in a pot of cold water. Bring water to a boil, then reduce heat and simmer for 12 minutes. Add cabbage and boil until barely soft. Add spinach and boil another minute until barely wilted and still a bright green color. Drain vegetables immediately into a colander and refresh by rinsing briefly with cold running water. Put 1 1/4 cups fresh water in the pot and bring to a boil. Turn heat to low and add tofu cubes.

Break the Udon noodles into thirds and cook according to the package instructions. Add cooked noodles to the tofu pot.

Whisk thoroughly or blend in a blender 1/2 cup of the water from the tofu pot and the raw tahini, miso, tamari sauce, and sesame oil with garlic and onion powder to taste. (Tahini, miso, tamari and Udon noodles are available in grocery stores.) Add to the tofu pot along with the drained mushrooms, spinach and cabbage. Add a slight pinch of hot pepper to taste. Reheat, being careful not to boil the soup. Serve hot.

	Saturated Calories	Mono & Poly Calories	Protein Calories	Carb Calories	Total Calories	Cholesterol (mg)
DAY 12						
Breakfast						
1 oz shredded wheat dry cereal	0	5	9	88	102	0
with 1/3 cup low-fat milk	2	3	11	18	34	3
3 stewed prunes toppped	0	0	1	53	54	0
with 2 tsp. safflower margarine	7	61	0	0	68	0
Scant 1.5 oz. turkey sausage	20	33	31	0	84	34
cooked in a dab of safflower margarine	1	5	0	0	6	0
Noncaloric beverage	0	0	0	0	0	0
TOTALS	30	107	52	159	348	37
Total proportions	9%	31%	15%	45%		
Lunch						
♦ White bean and cabbage soup:						
2/3 cup cooked small white beans	2	3	49	135	189	0
1/2 cup cabbage	0	0	1	7	8	0
1/4 cup celery	0	0	0	3	3	0
1/4 cup carrots	0	0	1	14	15	0
1/4 cup onion	0	0	1	12	13	0
sautéed in 2 tsp. safflower oil	7	74	0	0	81	0
1/4 cup canned tomatoes	0	5	2	18	25	0
1 Tbsp. lemon juice	0	0	0	2	2	0
1 Tbsp. brown sugar	0	0	0	35	35	0
1 cup chicken broth (or more, if needed)	3	7	5	6	21	0
1/4 tsp. caraway seed, thyme, spices to taste	0	1	1	5	7	0
22 dry-roasted almonds	0	120	23	13	156	0
Noncaloric beverage	0	0	0	0	0	0
TOTALS	12	210	83	250	555	0
Total proportions	2%	38%	15%	45%		

♦   Before you make this hearty soup, it is best to soak the beans overnight in cold water and drain before preparing.

	Saturated Calories	Mono & Poly Calories	Protein Calories	Carb Calories	Total Calories	Cholesterol (mg)

Dinner

	Saturated Calories	Mono & Poly Calories	Protein Calories	Carb Calories	Total Calories	Cholesterol (mg)
3.5 oz. slice of lean meat loaf (ground beef)	65	100	96	52	313	108
with 1/4 cup onion	0	0	1	12	13	0
sautéed in 1 tsp. safflower margarine until slightly burnt	3	34	0	0	37	0
and topped with 1 Tbsp. tomato sauce	0	1	1	15	17	0
1/2 cup cauliflower	0	1	4	10	15	0
with 2 tsp. safflower margarine	7	61	0	0	68	0
1 cup boiled collard greens with lemon juice	0	1	7	20	28	0
and 1 tsp. diced Canadian bacon	1	3	6	0	10	0
1 cup new potatoes	1	2	19	204	226	0
with 2 tsp. olive oil and spices	11	71	0	0	82	0
Scant 1/2 cup strawberry sorbet	0	0	2	95	97	0
Noncaloric beverage	0	0	0	0	0	0
TOTALS	88	274	136	408	906	108
Total proportions	10%	30%	15%	45%		

DAY 13

Breakfast

	Saturated Calories	Mono & Poly Calories	Protein Calories	Carb Calories	Total Calories	Cholesterol (mg)
1 large toasted bagel	0	16	24	122	162	0
with 2 1/2 tsp. safflower margarine	9	78	0	0	87	0
and 4 tsp. light cream cheese	12	12	10	5	39	10
mixed with 1 heaping tsp. low-fat cottage cheese	8	7	14	3	32	1
1/2 cup apple slices	0	0	0	30	30	0
Noncaloric beverage	0	0	0	0	0	0
TOTALS	29	113	48	160	350	11
Total proportions	8%	32%	14%	46%		

Lunch

	Saturated Calories	Mono & Poly Calories	Protein Calories	Carb Calories	Total Calories	Cholesterol (mg)
♦ Hungarian beef stew:						
2 oz. lean sirloin	17	28	64	0	109	22
2 tsp. canola oil	7	75	0	0	82	0
½ clove garlic, spices and						
1 Tbsp. beef broth	0	0	2	1	3	1
1 Tbsp. onion	0	0	0	3	3	0
1 tsp. balsamic vinegar	0	0	0	0	0	0
1 small Romano tomato	0	1	1	14	16	0
½ large potato	0	0	6	81	87	0
⅓ cup boiled celery root	0	1	2	17	20	0
½ cup shredded carrot	0	0	3	32	35	0
½ cup cucumber slices	0	0	1	6	7	0
1 oz. julienne beets	0	0	4	22	26	0
separately marinated in						
1 tsp. each of vinaigrette						
(4 tsp. total)	0	92	0	2	94	0
with 3 tomato wedges	0	1	3	14	18	
on 1 cup butter lettuce	0	1	1	8	10	0
1 small apple	0	0	0	50	50	0
Noncaloric beverage	0	0	0	0	0	0
TOTALS	24	199	87	250	560	23
Total proportions	4%	36%	15%	45%		

♦ Cut the meat into 1-inch cubes. Pat dry with toweling and sprinkle with salt. Put the oil into a skillet. When the pan is hot, brown all sides of the meat, turning frequently. Transfer the meat to a Dutch oven or large pot with a lid. Add beef broth, onion, tomato, garlic and bay leaf. Cover and simmer for 1½ hours or longer, stirring occasionally. Add more beef broth or water as necessary to prevent the stew from burning. Remove bay leaf and garlic clove. Add the cubed potato and simmer another 30 minutes or until potatoes are done. Add the balsamic vinegar and salt to taste. Thicken with 1 teaspoon flour, if desired. Variation: add parsley, carrots and peas.

Dinner

	Saturated Calories	Mono & Poly Calories	Protein Calories	Carb Calories	Total Calories	Cholesterol (mg)
♦ Seared scallops and fettuccini: 4 oz. fresh scallops	1	7	77	11	96	38
sautéed in 1 generous Tbsp. olive oil and 1 tsp. garlic	23	155	0	0	178	0

	Saturated Calories	Mono & Poly Calories	Protein Calories	Carb Calories	Total Calories	Cholesterol (mg)
with 1 tsp. parsley	0	0	0	1	1	0
pinch of dry red pepper flakes	0	0	0	1	1	0
1 tsp. capers and spices to taste	0	0	0	2	2	0
3 oz. fettuccini or spaghetti noodles	0	15	43	256	314	0
1 slice garlic bread	0	9	12	48	69	0
made with 1 Tbsp. safflower margarine	11	91	0	0	102	0
1 cup mixed baby greens	0	0	0	2	2	0
with 2 tsp. vinaigrette	9	39	0	1	49	0
1/2 small guava	0	1	2	45	48	0
and 1 sliced fresh peach	0	2	1	36	39	0
Noncaloric beverage	0	0	0	0	0	0
TOTALS	44	319	135	403	901	38
Total proportions	5%	35%	15%	45%		

♦ Rinse scallops in cold water and dry gently and thoroughly with toweling. Cut into $3/8$-inch pieces. Put the olive oil and 1 teaspoon minced garlic into a saucepan and sauté until light golden. Add parsley, red pepper flakes and capers (optional) and stir. When adding the hot pepper, start with a pinch per serving and add more later, if desired. Turn the heat to high and when hot, add the scallops and salt to taste. Cook on high 1 minute, constantly stirring. When the scallops turn a flat white, remove them from the heat and set aside. Cook the fettuccini or spaghetti noodles until firm (al dente). Turn the heat up high again on the scallops for a few seconds to reheat them. Do not boil away the delicious liquid from the scallops. Serve over drained pasta.

DAY 14

Breakfast

1 cup melon balls	0	1	4	50	55	0
2 4-in. buttermilk pancakes	3	4	13	106	126	0
with 2 tsp. safflower margarine	7	61	0	0	68	0
2 oz. chicken apple sausage	20	38	34	0	92	38
Noncaloric beverage	0	0	0	0	0	0

	Saturated Calories	Mono & Poly Calories	Protein Calories	Carb Calories	Total Calories	Cholesterol (mg)
TOTALS	30	104	51	156	341	38
Total proportions	9%	31%	15%	45%		

Lunch

	Saturated Calories	Mono & Poly Calories	Protein Calories	Carb Calories	Total Calories	Cholesterol (mg)
1 cup black bean soup	3	13	20	81	117	0
6 asparagus spears wrapped in 2 slices	0	1	7	16	24	0
white-meat turkey drizzled with 1 Tbsp.	0	4	36	2	42	7
vinaigrette	9	62	0	1	72	0
2 slices French bread with 1 Tbsp. safflower	0	18	22	100	140	0
margarine	11	91	0	0	102	0
1 fig bar cookie	0	8	1	44	53	0
Noncaloric beverage	0	0	0	0	0	0
TOTALS	23	197	86	244	550	7
Total proportions	4%	36%	15%	45%		

Dinner

	Saturated Calories	Mono & Poly Calories	Protein Calories	Carb Calories	Total Calories	Cholesterol (mg)
♦ Linguini and clams: with 2.5 oz. canned clams	1	11	72	15	99	47
3 oz. linguini	0	15	43	256	314	0
1 Tbsp. olive oil	23	155	0	0	178	0
1 small clove garlic, 1 tsp. parsley, 1 tsp. roasted hot red peppers	0	0	0	2	2	0
2 generous slices garlic bread	0	20	24	128	172	0
made with 1 Tbsp. safflower margarine topping	11	91	0	0	102	0
2 cups mixed baby greens	0	0	0	4	4	0
with scant 2 tsp. vinaigrette	7	32	0	1	40	0
Noncaloric beverage	0	0	0	0	0	0
TOTALS	42	324	139	406	911	47
Total proportions	5%	35%	15%	45%		

♦ Drain clams thoroughly and set aside. Put the olive oil and minced garlic into a saucepan and sauté until light golden. Add parsley and a pinch of hot peppers (to taste). Add clams and salt to taste. Sauté for 30 to 40 seconds on medium-high heat. Serve over linguini, cooked firm to the bite (al dente).

	Saturated Calories	Mono & Poly Calories	Protein Calories	Carb Calories	Total Calories	Cholesterol (mg)

DAY 15

Breakfast

	Saturated Calories	Mono & Poly Calories	Protein Calories	Carb Calories	Total Calories	Cholesterol (mg)
½ cup cooked oatmeal with cinnamon	0	11	11	51	73	0
topped with 2 tsp. sliced almonds	1	24	1	4	30	0
⅓ cup low-fat milk	2	3	11	18	34	3
½ grapefruit	0	1	1	34	36	0
1 slice whole wheat toast	0	9	10	45	64	0
with 2 tsp. safflower margarine	7	61	0	0	68	0
1 slice Canadian bacon	7	12	19	4	42	13
Noncaloric beverage	0	0	0	0	0	0
TOTALS	17	121	53	156	347	16
Total proportions	5%	35%	15%	45%		

Lunch

	Saturated Calories	Mono & Poly Calories	Protein Calories	Carb Calories	Total Calories	Cholesterol (mg)
Baked sesame burger: 1 store-bought tofu cake	8	45	45	13	111	0
sprinkled with 1 scant Tbsp. sunflower seeds	4	33	9	10	56	0
and 2 tsp. toasted sesame seeds	2	16	5	2	25	0
Garnish with alfalfa sprouts	0	0	2	3	5	0
and tamari sauce	0	0	0	10	10	0
mixed with 2 tsp. tahini dressing	6	42	7	8	63	0
on 1 hamburger bun	0	20	10	82	112	0
2 cups mixed baby greens	0	0	0	4	4	0
cucumber slices	0	0	0	2	2	0
3 tomato wedges	0	0	0	4	4	0
2 tsp. Raspberry vinaigrette	0	45	0	1	46	0
3 medium fresh figs	0	5	4	112	121	0

	Saturated Calories	Mono & Poly Calories	Protein Calories	Carb Calories	Total Calories	Cholesterol (mg)
Noncaloric beverage	0	0	0	0	0	0
TOTALS	20	206	82	251	559	0
Total proportions	4%	36%	15%	45%		

Dinner

	Saturated Calories	Mono & Poly Calories	Protein Calories	Carb Calories	Total Calories	Cholesterol (mg)
4.5 oz. lean baked ham	17	36	96	0	149	49
½ cup yams	0	1	5	76	82	0
with 2 tsp. safflower margarine	7	61	0	0	68	0
½ cup green beans	0	2	4	21	27	0
½ cup brussels sprouts	1	3	9	28	41	0
with 2 tsp. safflower margarine	7	61	0	0	68	0
⅓ generous cup mashed potato	7	23	12	108	150	2
with 1 tsp. safflower margarine	3	34	0	0	37	0
1 slice apple pie (⅛ of a pie)	21	86	10	172	289	0
Noncaloric beverage	0	0	0	0	0	0
TOTALS	63	307	136	405	911	51
Total proportions	7%	33%	15%	45%		

DAY 16

Breakfast

	Saturated Calories	Mono & Poly Calories	Protein Calories	Carb Calories	Total Calories	Cholesterol (mg)
4 oz. fresh orange juice	0	0	3	52	55	0
1 oat bran English muffin	0	11	19	98	128	0
with 2 generous tsp. safflower margarine	8	66	0	0	74	3
1.5 oz. turkey sausage	20	33	37	0	90	34
Noncaloric beverage	0	0	0	0	0	0
TOTALS	28	110	59	150	347	37
Total proportions	8%	32%	17%	43%		

	Saturated Calories	Mono & Poly Calories	Protein Calories	Carb Calories	Total Calories	Cholesterol (mg)
Lunch						
Picnic with 1.75 oz. chicken breast (fried in safflower oil)	11	30	61	5	107	47
½ cup potato salad made with safflower mayo, oil and vinegar	8	95	3	54	160	0
2 biscuits (from mix)	0	60	16	105	181	0
1 slice watermelon (1 cup)	0	5	4	48	57	0
1 small chocolate mint	4	7	0	38	49	0
Noncaloric beverage	0	0	0	0	0	0
TOTALS	23	197	84	250	554	47
Total proportions	4%	36%	15%	45%		
Dinner						
Scant 5 oz. fresh crab	1	7	95	3	106	52
dipped in 2 Tbsp. melted safflower margarine mixed with lemon juice to taste	20	176	2	2	200	0
½ cup cooked spinach with spices and 1 tsp.	0	2	10	14	26	0
safflower margarine	3	34	0	0	37	0
1 large baked potato	0	2	21	247	270	0
with 2 tsp. chives	0	0	0	1	1	0
and generous 2 tsp. safflower margarine	8	72	0	0	80	0
3-in. square gingerbread (from mix)	0	36	8	143	187	0
Noncaloric beverage	0	0	0	0	0	0
TOTALS	32	329	136	410	907	52
Total proportions	4%	36%	15%	45%		

DAY 17

Breakfast

	Saturated Calories	Mono & Poly Calories	Protein Calories	Carb Calories	Total Calories	Cholesterol (mg)
¾ cup raisin bran dry cereal	0	6	16	93	115	0
with ⅓ cup low-fat milk	2	3	11	18	34	3

	Saturated Calories	Mono & Poly Calories	Protein Calories	Carb Calories	Total Calories	Cholesterol (mg)
1 slice Canadian bacon	7	12	19	4	42	13
1 slice rye toast	0	8	9	49	66	0
with 1 Tbsp. safflower margarine	11	91	0	0	102	0
Noncaloric beverage	0	0	0	0	0	0
TOTALS	20	120	55	164	359	16
Total proportions	6%	34%	15%	45%		

Lunch

	Saturated Calories	Mono & Poly Calories	Protein Calories	Carb Calories	Total Calories	Cholesterol (mg)
Crab sandwich: 2 oz. crabmeat	0	2	42	0	44	23
with 5½ tsp. safflower mayo	14	156	4	7	181	0
chopped celery and 1 lettuce leaf	0	0	0	2	2	0
on 1 sourdough roll	0	20	24	96	140	0
1 medium artichoke drizzled with lemon juice	0	2	11	50	63	0
1 cup cooked squash with wine and Worcestershire sauce	0	4	6	35	45	0
5 vanilla wafers	0	25	1	60	86	0
Noncaloric beverage	0	0	0	0	0	0
TOTALS	14	209	88	250	561	23
Total proportions	3%	37%	15%	45%		

Dinner

	Saturated Calories	Mono & Poly Calories	Protein Calories	Carb Calories	Total Calories	Cholesterol (mg)
½ small chicken breast	15	40	89	5	149	88
fried in safflower oil	10	110	0	0	120	0
1 cup mashed potato	9	30	15	143	197	2
with 2 tsp. safflower margarine	7	61	0	0	68	0
½ cup green beans	0	2	4	21	27	0
½ cup cucumber, carrots and radish	0	1	1	7	9	0
Corn on the cob (½ cup)	2	8	10	84	104	0
with 2 tsp. safflower margarine	7	61	0	0	68	0

	Saturated Calories	Mono & Poly Calories	Protein Calories	Carb Calories	Total Calories	Cholesterol (mg)
1 slice angel food cake (unfrosted)	0	0	17	144	161	0
Noncaloric beverage	0	0	0	0	0	0
TOTALS	50	313	136	404	903	90
Total proportions	5%	35%	15%	45%		

DAY 18

Breakfast

	Saturated Calories	Mono & Poly Calories	Protein Calories	Carb Calories	Total Calories	Cholesterol (mg)
½ cup cooked cream of wheat	0	2	8	57	67	0
with 1½ tsp. safflower margarine	5	45	0	0	50	0
1 cup fresh strawberries	0	1	2	42	45	0
1 slice whole wheat toast	0	9	10	45	64	0
with 2 tsp. safflower margarine	7	61	0	0	68	0
¼ cup low-fat cottage cheese	4	3	31	8	46	5
Noncaloric beverage	0	0	0	0	0	0
TOTALS	16	121	51	152	340	5
Total proportions	5%	35%	15%	45%		

Lunch

	Saturated Calories	Mono & Poly Calories	Protein Calories	Carb Calories	Total Calories	Cholesterol (mg)
Grilled fillet of sole (medium to small)	0	5	56	2	63	0
with 2 Tbsp. tartar sauce	0	160	0	0	160	0
and 1 tomato slice	0	0	1	5	6	0
on 1 roll	0	19	13	81	113	0
4 wedges roasted red potato	0	1	11	136	148	0
drizzled with 2 tsp. rosemary olive oil	4	36	0	0	40	0
1 ladyfinger cookie	1	6	6	30	43	0
Noncaloric beverage	0	0	0	0	0	0
TOTALS	5	227	87	254	573	0
Total proportions	1%	39%	15%	45%		

	Saturated Calories	Mono & Poly Calories	Protein Calories	Carb Calories	Total Calories	Cholesterol (mg)
Dinner						
3 oz. lean roasted lamb	30	33	90	0	153	0
½ cup macaroni and cheese	54	93	33	81	261	0
½ cup brussels sprouts with 2 tsp. safflower margarine	1 7	3 61	8 0	28 0	40 68	0 0
½ cup cooked carrots with 1½ tsp. safflower margarine	0 4	1 45	3 0	33 0	37 49	0 0
1 cup mandarin orange sorbet	0	2	4	224	230	0
2 refrigerator-dough sugar cookies	0	30	1	40	71	0
Noncaloric beverage	0	0	0	0	0	0
TOTALS	96	268	139	406	909	0
Total proportions	10%	30%	15%	45%		

DAY 19

Breakfast

1 oz. shredded wheat dry cereal	0	5	9	88	102	0
with ⅓ cup low-fat milk	2	3	11	18	34	3
3 stewed prunes topped with 2 tsp. safflower margarine	0 7	0 61	1 0	53 0	54 68	0 0
Scant 1.5 oz. turkey sausage cooked in a dab of safflower margarine	20 1	33 5	31 0	0 0	84 6	34 0
Noncaloric beverage	0	0	0	0	0	0
TOTALS	30	107	52	159	348	37
Total proportions	5%	35%	15%	45%		

Lunch

2 oz. lean grilled hamburger	36	57	62	0	155	58
with 1 tsp. mustard	0	1	1	2	4	0

	Saturated Calories	Mono & Poly Calories	Protein Calories	Carb Calories	Total Calories	Cholesterol (mg)
and 1 Tbsp. catsup	0	1	1	14	16	0
on 1 bun	0	20	12	82	114	0
1 small/medium sliced tomato	0	2	2	10	14	0
3 cucumber sticks	0	0	1	6	7	0
drizzled with ½ Tbsp. vinaigrette	2	35	0	1	38	0
10 Greek olives	5	55	1	4	65	0
5 radishes	0	1	1	3	5	0
1 large banana	1	3	5	131	140	0
Noncaloric beverage	0	0	0	0	0	0
TOTALS	44	175	86	253	558	58
Total proportions	8%	32%	15%	45%		

Dinner

	Saturated Calories	Mono & Poly Calories	Protein Calories	Carb Calories	Total Calories	Cholesterol (mg)
3.25 oz. turkey summer sausage	35	67	61	6	169	123
fried in 1 tsp. safflower oil	3	36	0	0	39	0
♦ ¾ red cabbage	0	3	5	21	29	0
⅓ cup beef broth	1	1	2	3	7	0
1 tsp. safflower margarine	3	31	0	0	34	0
1 to 2 tsp. balsamic vinegar	0	0	0	1	1	0
1 slice Canadian bacon, diced	7	25	47	0	79	4
½ tart green apple, sliced	0	2	1	42	45	0
1 tsp. brown sugar	0	0	0	12	12	0
1 cup garlic mashed potatoes	20	59	16	140	235	3
with 2 tsp. safflower margarine	8	60	0	0	68	0
Generous ¾ cup applesauce	0	3	1	178	182	0
Noncaloric beverage	0	0	0	0	0	0
TOTALS	77	287	133	403	900	130
Total proportions	8%	32%	15%	45%		

♦ To prepare the red cabbage, shred the cabbage after removing the hard core. Soak cabbage for a few minutes in cold water. Drain and add beef broth, margarine, vinegar, Canadian bacon, brown sugar and apple. Cook on low heat until apples are soft and blended with the cabbage. Add salt and spices to taste.

DAY 20

	Saturated Calories	Mono & Poly Calories	Protein Calories	Carb Calories	Total Calories	Cholesterol (mg)
Breakfast						
1 large toasted bagel	0	16	24	122	162	0
with 2½ tsp. safflower margarine	9	78	0	0	87	0
and 4 tsp. light cream cheese	12	12	10	5	39	10
mixed with 1 heaping Tbsp. low-fat cottage cheese	8	7	14	3	32	1
½ cup apple slices	0	0	0	30	30	0
Noncaloric beverage	0	0	0	0	0	0
TOTALS	29	113	48	160	350	11
Total proportions	8%	32%	14%	46%		
Lunch						
Chicken and biscuits:						
2 oz. stewed chicken	9	26	62	0	97	56
with ¼ cup celery	0	0	0	3	3	0
¼ cup carrots	0	0	1	14	15	0
¼ cup onion	0	0	1	12	13	0
¼ cubed potato	0	1	2	24	27	0
and spices to taste (clove, allspice, bay leaf)	0	0	1	7	8	0
2 biscuits (from mix)	0	60	16	105	181	0
1 Tbsp. safflower margarine	11	91	0	0	102	0
1 oz. chocolate fudge	10	20	3	86	119	0
Noncaloric beverage	0	0	0	0	0	0
TOTALS	30	198	86	251	565	56
Total proportions	5%	35%	15%	45%		
Dinner						
3.25 oz. trout	11	52	88	0	151	61
dusted in 2 Tbsp. flour	0	1	8	53	62	0
and fried in 1 Tbsp. safflower oil (leaving oil residue in pan)	10	110	0	0	120	0

	Saturated Calories	Mono & Poly Calories	Protein Calories	Carb Calories	Total Calories	Cholesterol (mg)
6 large asparagus spears with scant 1 tsp. safflower margarine and	1	2	10	21	34	0
1 tsp. lemon juice	2	24	0	0	26	0
½ cup corn on the cob with 1 tsp. safflower	2	8	12	84	106	0
margarine	3	34	0	0	37	0
1 large baked potato with 1 Tbsp. safflower	0	2	21	247	270	0
margarine	11	91	0	0	102	0
Noncaloric beverage	0	0	0	0	0	0
TOTALS	40	324	139	405	908	61
Total proportions	4%	36%	15%	45%		

DAY 21

Breakfast

	Saturated Calories	Mono & Poly Calories	Protein Calories	Carb Calories	Total Calories	Cholesterol (mg)
1 cup melon balls	0	1	4	50	55	0
2 4-in. buttermilk pancakes with 2 tsp. safflower	3	4	13	106	126	0
margarine	7	61	0	0	68	0
2 oz. chicken apple sausage	20	38	34	0	92	38
Noncaloric beverage	0	0	0	0	0	0
TOTALS	30	104	51	156	341	38
Total proportions	8%	31%	15%	45%		

Lunch

	Saturated Calories	Mono & Poly Calories	Protein Calories	Carb Calories	Total Calories	Cholesterol (mg)
3 oz. grilled sea bass on a sourdough roll with 1 Tbsp. tartar sauce, lettuce and tomato	3	109	79	100	291	35
½ cup potato salad made with safflower mayo and oil and vinegar	9	95	3	53	160	0
3 fresh apricots	0	2	2	47	51	0
2 dried dates	0	0	1	49	50	0

	Saturated Calories	Mono & Poly Calories	Protein Calories	Carb Calories	Total Calories	Cholesterol (mg)
Noncaloric beverage	0	0	0	0	0	0
TOTALS	12	206	85	249	552	35
Total proportions	2%	38%	15%	45%		

Dinner

	Saturated Calories	Mono & Poly Calories	Protein Calories	Carb Calories	Total Calories	Cholesterol (mg)
Beans and franks: 1 turkey frank	22	57	23	37	139	45
on a hot dog bun	0	19	14	81	114	0
with 1 Tbsp. mustard	0	8	4	4	16	0
and 1 Tbsp. catsup	0	1	1	14	16	0
1 cup baked beans	0	0	59	217	276	0
with 2 tsp. safflower margarine	7	61	0	0	68	0
1 artichoke	0	2	11	49	62	0
with 1⅓ Tbsp. safflower mayo mixed with lemon to taste	14	117	1	2	134	0
1 cup mixed baby greens	0	0	0	2	2	0
with 1 oz. shrimp	1	4	23	1	29	43
and 2 tsp. vinaigrette	9	39	0	1	49	0
Noncaloric beverage	0	0	0	0	0	0
TOTALS	53	308	136	408	905	88
Total proportions	6%	34%	15%	45%		

DAY 22

Breakfast

	Saturated Calories	Mono & Poly Calories	Protein Calories	Carb Calories	Total Calories	Cholesterol (mg)
½ cup cooked oatmeal with cinnamon	0	11	11	51	73	0
topped with 2 tsp. sliced almonds	1	24	1	4	30	0
⅓ cup low-fat milk	2	3	11	18	34	3
½ grapefruit	0	1	1	34	36	0
1 slice whole wheat toast	0	9	10	45	64	0
with 2 tsp. safflower margarine	7	61	0	0	68	0
1 slice Canadian bacon	7	12	19	4	42	13

	Saturated Calories	Mono & Poly Calories	Protein Calories	Carb Calories	Total Calories	Cholesterol (mg)
Noncaloric beverage	0	0	0	0	0	0
TOTALS	17	121	53	156	347	16
Total proportions	5%	35%	15%	45%		

Lunch

	Saturated Calories	Mono & Poly Calories	Protein Calories	Carb Calories	Total Calories	Cholesterol (mg)
Chicken burrito:						
1 oz. chicken breast	3	8	32	0	43	24
with ¼ cup rice	0	0	3	50	53	0
and ¾ cup refried beans with 2 tsp. olive oil	17	80	45	140	282	0
rolled in 1 small flour tortilla	0	18	7	50	75	0
1 cup fresh cabbage coleslaw	0	0	1	15	16	0
with 1 Tbsp. safflower mayo	11	88	0	1	100	0
Noncaloric beverage	0	0	0	0	0	0
TOTALS	31	194	88	256	569	24
Total proportions	5%	35%	15%	45%		

Dinner

	Saturated Calories	Mono & Poly Calories	Protein Calories	Carb Calories	Total Calories	Cholesterol (mg)
2.5 oz. roasted pheasant without skin	8	16	66	0	90	0
1 cup cooked wild and long-grain rice mix	43	31	21	198	293	10
with 1 Tbsp. toasted filbert nuts	0	65	11	10	86	0
and ¼ cup burnt diced onion	0	0	1	12	13	0
sautéed in 2 tsp. safflower oil	8	74	0	0	82	0
♦ ¾ cup red cabbage	0	3	5	21	29	0
⅓ cup beef broth	1	1	2	3	7	0
1 to 2 tsp. balsamic vinegar	0	0	0	1	1	0
½ slice Canadian bacon	3	14	22	0	39	0
½ tart green apple, sliced	0	2	1	42	45	0
1 tsp. brown sugar	0	0	0	12	12	0
6 asparagus spears	1	2	9	16	28	0
topped with 2½ generous tsp. safflower margarine and 1 tsp. lemon juice	10	80	0	0	90	0
Scant ½ cup lemon sorbet	0	1	1	92	94	0

	Saturated Calories	Mono & Poly Calories	Protein Calories	Carb Calories	Total Calories	Cholesterol (mg)
Noncaloric beverage	0	0	0	0	0	0
TOTALS	74	289	139	407	909	10
Total proportions	8%	32%	15%	45%		

♦ Prepare the red cabbage according to the instructions for this recipe on Day 19 at the 1,200 calorie diet (p. 201), leaving out the margarine.

DAY 23

Breakfast

	Saturated Calories	Mono & Poly Calories	Protein Calories	Carb Calories	Total Calories	Cholesterol (mg)
4 oz. fresh orange juice	0	0	3	52	55	0
1 oat bran English muffin	0	11	19	98	128	0
with 2 generous tsp. safflower margarine	8	66	0	0	74	3
1.5 oz. turkey sausage	20	33	37	0	90	34
Noncaloric beverage	0	0	0	0	0	0
TOTALS	28	110	59	150	347	37
Total proportions	8%	32%	17%	43%		

Lunch

	Saturated Calories	Mono & Poly Calories	Protein Calories	Carb Calories	Total Calories	Cholesterol (mg)
♦ Cheese-baked tofu: ½-in.-thick tofu slice sprinkled with garlic tamari sauce and 4 tsp.	10	27	50	14	101	0
grated Gruyère or Emmentaler cheese	35	20	16	1	72	20
♦ Curried rice: ½ cup cooked brown rice	0	11	10	99	120	0
with onion and garlic	0	0	0	3	3	0
1 Tbsp. zucchini	0	0	0	2	2	0
1 mushroom	0	1	1	4	6	0
mung bean sprouts	0	0	2	6	8	0
sautéed in 1 Tbsp. safflower oil	10	110	0	0	120	0
1 large pear	0	0	4	120	124	0

	Saturated Calories	Mono & Poly Calories	Protein Calories	Carb Calories	Total Calories	Cholesterol (mg)
Noncaloric beverage	0	0	0	0	0	0
TOTALS	55	169	83	249	556	20
Total proportions	10%	30%	15%	45%		

♦ To prepare the tofu, preheat the oven to 350° and coat a baking tray or dish with nonstick baking spray. Set aside. Poke holes in the tofu patty with a fork and sprinkle with garlic tamari sauce. (Tamari sauce is a light and flavorful soy-based sauce that can be found in many grocery stores, especially those that stock Japanese food products.) Sprinkle the cheeses on the patty and bake until a bit crusty, or about 20 minutes.

Prepare the rice according to the directions on the package. Remove from heat and keep covered. Heat oil in a skillet over medium heat. Add 1 tablespoon onion. When the onion is light golden, add 1/2 chopped clove garlic and sauté until the onion is slightly burnt. Add the zucchini, chopped mushroom and 1 tablespoon mung bean sprouts. Add 1/4 teaspoon curry powder (or to taste). Cook, stirring frequently, for 5 minutes on medium heat. Fluff the rice with a fork and add to the skillet. Cook and stir frequently for 2 to 3 minutes. Serve.

Dinner

	Saturated Calories	Mono & Poly Calories	Protein Calories	Carb Calories	Total Calories	Cholesterol (mg)
♦ Stir-fried vegetables and noodles: 1/4 onion	0	1	2	12	15	0
in 1 Tbsp. safflower oil	10	110	0	0	120	0
1 shredded red chili	0	1	4	17	22	0
1/2 peeled, shredded carrot	0	0	1	15	16	0
1/2 cup bean sprouts	0	1	3	3	7	0
garlic, spices and 1 Tbsp. soy sauce	0	0	1	5	6	0
1 cup cooked rice noodles or spaghetti noodles	0	14	14	130	158	0
2 oz. grilled swordfish	5	15	44	0	64	22
on 1 roll	0	19	11	72	102	0
1 teaspoon tartar sauce	0	35	0	0	35	0
1 cup custard	61	70	57	118	306	110
3 vanilla wafers	0	15	1	36	52	0
Noncaloric beverage	0	0	0	0	0	0
TOTALS	76	281	138	408	903	132
Total proportions	8%	32%	15%	45%		

♦ To prepare the stir-fried vegetables, heat the oil on medium-high heat in a skillet and add the chopped onion, red chili, carrot and bean sprouts. Sauté with a dash of garlic powder or half a clove of fresh minced garlic, salt to taste and soy sauce, until done firm to the bite (al dente). Serve over the noodles.

	Saturated Calories	Mono & Poly Calories	Protein Calories	Carb Calories	Total Calories	Cholesterol (mg)

DAY 24

Breakfast

	Saturated Calories	Mono & Poly Calories	Protein Calories	Carb Calories	Total Calories	Cholesterol (mg)
¾ cup raisin bran dry cereal	0	6	16	93	115	0
with ⅓ cup low-fat milk	2	3	11	18	34	3
1 slice Canadian bacon	7	12	19	4	42	13
1 slice rye toast	0	8	9	49	66	0
with 1 Tbsp. safflower margarine	11	91	0	0	102	0
Noncaloric beverage	0	0	0	0	0	0
TOTALS	20	120	55	164	359	16
Total proportions	6%	34%	15%	45%		

Lunch

	Saturated Calories	Mono & Poly Calories	Protein Calories	Carb Calories	Total Calories	Cholesterol (mg)
Shrimp burrito: 1 oz. shrimp	1	5	23	1	30	43
⅔ cup refried beans with 2 tsp. olive oil	16	79	42	125	262	0
1 flour tortilla	0	18	9	60	87	0
8 tortilla chips	0	9	8	51	68	0
1 cup cabbage coleslaw	0	0	1	15	16	0
with 1 Tbsp. safflower mayo	11	88	0	1	100	0
Noncaloric beverage	0	0	0	0	0	0
TOTALS	28	199	83	253	563	43
Total proportions	5%	35%	15%	45%		

	Saturated Calories	Mono & Poly Calories	Protein Calories	Carb Calories	Total Calories	Cholesterol (mg)
Dinner						
2.75 oz. roasted Cornish game hen (without skin)	14	39	90	0	143	69
basted in 1 tsp. olive oil	5	35	0	0	40	0
and stuffed with 1 cup cooked wild and long-grain rice	43	31	21	198	293	10
1 Tbsp. filbert nuts	0	65	11	10	86	0
1/4 cup burnt diced onion	0	0	1	12	13	0
sautéed in 1 tsp. safflower oil	4	37	0	0	41	0
2 Tbsp. currant jelly	0	0	0	51	51	0
1 artichoke	0	2	11	50	63	0
dipped in lemon juice with 2 1/2 tsp. melted safflower margarine	9	77	0	0	86	0
1/3 cup green beans	0	1	3	13	17	0
1/3 cup peach sorbet	0	0	1	78	79	0
Noncaloric beverage	0	0	0	0	0	0
TOTALS	75	287	138	412	912	79
Total proportions	8%	32%	15%	45%		

DAY 25

	Saturated Calories	Mono & Poly Calories	Protein Calories	Carb Calories	Total Calories	Cholesterol (mg)
1/2 cup cooked cream of wheat	0	2	8	57	67	0
with 1 1/2 tsp. safflower margarine	5	45	0	0	50	0
1 cup fresh strawberries	0	1	2	42	45	0
1 slice whole wheat toast	0	9	10	45	64	0
with 2 tsp. safflower margarine	7	61	0	0	68	0
1/4 cup low-fat cottage cheese	4	3	31	8	46	5
Noncaloric beverage	0	0	0	0	0	0
TOTALS	16	121	51	152	340	5
Total proportions	5%	35%	15%	45%		

	Saturated Calories	Mono & Poly Calories	Protein Calories	Carb Calories	Total Calories	Cholesterol (mg)
Lunch						
1¼ cups spaghetti, meatballs and tomato sauce	19	78	72	158	327	15
1 cup green salad with ¼ cup broccoli, ½ oz. croutons, cucumbers, carrots, tomato slices	0	22	8	56	86	0
2 Tbsp. oil and vinegar dressing	0	104	0	4	108	0
3 chocolate snap cookies	0	0	2	34	36	0
Noncaloric beverage	0	0	0	0	0	0
TOTALS	19	204	82	252	557	15
Total proportions	3%	37%	15%	45%		
Dinner						
♦ Curried lamb:						
2.75 oz. lean lamb with fat trimmed	28	22	88	0	138	0
¼ cup onion	0	0	1	12	13	0
garlic, lemon juice, curry spices	0	4	1	5	10	0
3 Tbsp. yogurt	8	4	6	8	26	5
2 tsp. safflower margarine	7	61	0	0	68	0
♦ 1 cup cooked white rice	0	2	16	198	216	0
with 2 tsp. safflower margarine	7	61	0	0	68	0
fresh grated ginger and ½ cup chicken broth	1	4	3	3	11	1
1 Tbsp. grated coconut	16	2	2	11	31	0
¼ cup yogurt	10	6	7	10	33	6
with dash of cayenne pepper, cumin, salt, sugar	0	0	1	6	7	0
and shallots	0	0	0	11	11	0
mixed with ½ cup shredded cucumber	0	0	1	6	7	0
1 cup mixed vegetables with turmeric seasoning: onion, precooked potato, peas, parboiled cabbage, cauliflower, tomato and spinach	0	2	10	123	135	0

	Saturated Calories	Mono & Poly Calories	Protein Calories	Carb Calories	Total Calories	Cholesterol (mg)
sautéed in 1 generous Tbsp. safflower margarine	12	103	0	0	115	0
Noncaloric beverage	0	0	0	0	0	0
TOTALS	89	271	136	393	889	12
Total proportions	10%	30%	15%	45%		

♦ Lamb curry: Thoroughly dry the lamb with toweling. Put 1 teaspoon margarine into a heavy skillet on high heat. When hot, add 1-inch cubes of trimmed lamb and brown them on all sides. Set aside in a bowl. Add another teaspoon margarine and the onion to the skillet and reduce to medium-high heat. Sauté until the onion is slightly burnt (dark brown color), stirring frequently. Add garlic and 1 teaspoon chopped or grated fresh ginger, and sauté for another minute. Add $1/4$ to $1/2$ teaspoon curry powder and salt to taste and cook for an additional 10 to 15 seconds. Remove from the heat and immediately mix in $1/4$ cup yogurt. Add lamb and lemon juice to taste.

Coconut rice: Boil $1/2$ cup chicken broth per serving and add margarine. When the broth is boiling, add the rice. Add a pinch of fresh grated ginger and the grated coconut. Cover and cook according to the directions on the rice package. When done, let it rest for about 5 minutes before serving alongside the curry.

DAY 26

Breakfast

1 oz. shredded wheat dry cereal	0	5	9	88	102	0
with $1/3$ cup low-fat milk	2	3	11	18	34	3
3 stewed prunes	0	0	1	53	54	0
topped with 2 tsp. safflower margarine	7	61	0	0	68	0
Scant 1.5 oz. turkey sausage	20	33	31	0	84	34
cooked in a dab of safflower margarine	1	5	0	0	6	0
Noncaloric beverage	0	0	0	0	0	0
TOTALS	30	107	52	159	348	37
Total proportions	9%	31%	15%	45%		

	Saturated Calories	Mono & Poly Calories	Protein Calories	Carb Calories	Total Calories	Cholesterol (mg)

Lunch

	Saturated Calories	Mono & Poly Calories	Protein Calories	Carb Calories	Total Calories	Cholesterol (mg)
Caesar chicken salad:						
1 oz. chicken breast	4	10	40	0	54	85
3 cups romaine lettuce	0	0	2	9	11	0
lemon juice, wine vinegar, Worcestershire sauce, pepper and 1 Tbsp. garlic olive oil	16	104	0	0	120	0
2 Tbsp. Parmesan cheese	18	10	15	3	46	8
½ cup croutons	0	27	5	33	65	0
2 slices sourdough French bread	0	18	22	98	138	0
1 cup blackberries	0	1	1	74	76	0
with 1 small sugar cookie	0	12	1	33	46	0
Noncaloric beverage	0	0	0	0	0	0
TOTALS	38	182	86	250	556	93
Total proportions	7%	33%	15%	45%		

Dinner

	Saturated Calories	Mono & Poly Calories	Protein Calories	Carb Calories	Total Calories	Cholesterol (mg)
1 cup risotto (rice)	0	2	16	199	217	0
with 3.25 oz. shrimp	3	14	87	4	108	163
1 Tbsp. shallots	0	0	1	7	8	0
2 tsp. olive oil	9	71	0	0	80	0
2 tsp. grated Parmesan cheese	9	5	9	1	24	4
⅔ cup chicken broth	2	5	3	3	13	1
½ cup zucchini squash	0	2	5	16	23	0
with 2 tsp. safflower margarine	7	61	0	0	68	0
¾ cup four-bean salad	0	3	17	161	181	0
with 2 generous Tbsp. vinaigrette	0	169	0	0	169	0
Hot mint tea with 1 tsp. sugar	0	0	0	15	15	0
Noncaloric beverage	0	0	0	0	0	0
TOTALS	30	332	138	406	906	168
Total proportions	3%	37%	15%	45%		

	Saturated Calories	Mono & Poly Calories	Protein Calories	Carb Calories	Total Calories	Cholesterol (mg)

DAY 27

Breakfast

	Saturated Calories	Mono & Poly Calories	Protein Calories	Carb Calories	Total Calories	Cholesterol (mg)
1 large toasted bagel	0	16	24	122	162	0
with 2½ tsp. safflower margarine	9	78	0	0	87	0
and 4 tsp. light cream cheese	12	12	10	5	39	10
mixed with 1 heaping Tbsp. low-fat cottage cheese	8	7	14	3	32	1
½ cup apple slices	0	0	0	30	30	0
Noncaloric beverage	0	0	0	0	0	0
TOTALS	29	113	48	160	350	11
Total proportions	8%	32%	14%	46%		

Lunch

	Saturated Calories	Mono & Poly Calories	Protein Calories	Carb Calories	Total Calories	Cholesterol (mg)
1 grilled fillet of sole	0	3	70	2	75	0
20 french fries fried in safflower oil	43	104	12	160	319	0
1 small fresh papaya	1	2	3	80	86	0
sliced onto a bed of 4 romaine lettuce leaves drizzled with scant 1 Tbsp. honey vinaigrette	10	57	0	10	77	0
Noncaloric beverage	0	0	0	0	0	0
TOTALS	54	166	85	252	557	0
Total proportions	10%	30%	15%	45%		

Dinner

	Saturated Calories	Mono & Poly Calories	Protein Calories	Carb Calories	Total Calories	Cholesterol (mg)
3.5 oz. lean London broil marinated in 1 Tbsp. olive oil and red wine vinegar	57	77	100	0	234	70
(amount absorbed)	15	104	0	0	119	0
1 medium baked potato	1	1	19	204	225	0
with 2 tsp. safflower margarine	7	61	0	0	68	0

	Saturated Calories	Mono & Poly Calories	Protein Calories	Carb Calories	Total Calories	Cholesterol (mg)
½ cup small peas	0	0	17	50	67	0
with 1 Tbsp. onion	0	0	0	3	3	0
sautéed in scant 1 tsp. safflower margarine	2	30	0	0	32	0
1 cup fresh pineapple	0	6	2	77	85	0
on top of ⅓ cup pineapple or strawberry sorbet	0	0	1	74	75	0
Noncaloric beverage	0	0	0	0	0	0
TOTALS	82	279	139	408	908	70
Total proportions	9%	31%	15%	45%		

DAY 28

Breakfast

	Saturated Calories	Mono & Poly Calories	Protein Calories	Carb Calories	Total Calories	Cholesterol (mg)
1 cup melon balls	0	1	4	50	55	0
2 4-in. buttermilk pancakes	3	4	13	106	126	0
with 2 tsp. safflower margarine	7	61	0	0	68	0
2 oz. chicken apple sausage	20	38	34	0	92	38
Noncaloric beverage	0	0	0	0	0	0
TOTALS	30	104	51	156	341	38
Total proportions	9%	31%	15%	45%		

Lunch

	Saturated Calories	Mono & Poly Calories	Protein Calories	Carb Calories	Total Calories	Cholesterol (mg)
♦ Black bean chili:						
1 generous cup black beans cooked with chicken broth	2	7	70	194	273	0
and ¼ cup onion	0	0	1	12	13	0
¼ bell pepper	0	0	1	5	6	0
½ cup fresh tomato slices sautéed in generous	0	0	1	11	12	0
1½ Tbsp. safflower oil	16	180	0	0	196	0
1½ Tbsp. tomato paste	0	2	4	19	25	0
and ¼ tsp. each of oregano, cumin, paprika, coriander; ½ bay leaf, salt, pepper, ½ tsp. chili powder and						
1 tsp. red wine vinegar	0	0	2	8	10	0
topped with 4 tsp. Parmesan cheese	11	6	9	1	27	6

	Saturated Calories	Mono & Poly Calories	Protein Calories	Carb Calories	Total Calories	Cholesterol (mg)
Noncaloric beverage	0	0	0	0	0	0
TOTALS	29	195	88	250	562	6
Total proportions	5%	35%	15%	45%		

♦ Rinse the black beans and soak them overnight in cold water. Drain and rinse again. Add water to cover the beans, and 1 chicken bouillon cube per cup of water (or use canned chicken broth). Cook until tender, about 1¹/₂ hours. In a skillet, brown onion and bell pepper in safflower oil. Add onion and bell pepper to the beans. Add tomato and tomato paste, spices and vinegar. Cover and simmer another 1¹/₂ hours, adding chicken broth or water when needed. Serve topped with 4 teaspoons Parmesan cheese.

Dinner

	Saturated Calories	Mono & Poly Calories	Protein Calories	Carb Calories	Total Calories	Cholesterol (mg)
3 oz. halibut steak	4	19	89	0	112	35
baked crusty with equal mixture cornmeal and flour	0	0	2	10	12	0
and 1¹/₂ tsp. melted safflower margarine	5	45	0	0	50	0
1 cup cooked rice	0	2	16	199	217	0
with 2 Tbsp. pineapple	0	0	0	10	10	0
1 Tbsp. toasted pine nuts	12	66	7	11	96	0
¹/₂ cup green peas	0	2	15	50	67	0
with 1¹/₂ tsp. safflower margarine	5	45	0	0	50	0
1 small sweet potato	0	0	4	70	74	0
with 2 tsp. safflower margarine	7	61	0	0	68	0
1 dinner roll	0	19	9	56	84	0
with 2 tsp. safflower margarine	7	61	0	0	68	0
Noncaloric beverage	0	0	0	0	0	0
TOTALS	40	320	142	406	908	35
Total proportions	4%	36%	15%	45%		

DAY 29

Breakfast

	Saturated Calories	Mono & Poly Calories	Protein Calories	Carb Calories	Total Calories	Cholesterol (mg)
½ cup cooked oatmeal with cinnamon	0	11	11	51	73	0
topped with 2 tsp. sliced almonds	1	24	1	4	30	0
⅓ cup low-fat milk	2	3	11	18	34	3
½ grapefruit	0	1	1	34	36	0
1 slice whole wheat toast	0	9	10	45	64	0
with 2 tsp. safflower margarine	7	61	0	0	68	0
1 slice Canadian bacon	7	12	19	4	42	13
Noncaloric beverage	0	0	0	0	0	0
TOTALS	17	121	53	156	347	16
Total proportions	5%	35%	15%	45%		

Lunch

	Saturated Calories	Mono & Poly Calories	Protein Calories	Carb Calories	Total Calories	Cholesterol (mg)
Crab salad: 3 oz. crab	0	3	62	0	65	35
marinated in vinaigrette of 2½ tsp. Dijon mustard	0	5	2	2	9	0
1 Tbsp. minced shallots	0	0	1	6	7	0
2 tsp. white wine vinegar	0	0	0	1	1	0
1 Tbsp. olive oil	13	106	0	0	119	0
Set on 6 prebaked potato slices	2	3	20	240	265	0
sautéed in 2½ tsp. olive oil (leave residue in pan)	11	81	0	0	92	0
on bed of ½ cup fresh spinach	0	0	2	4	6	0
Noncaloric beverage	0	0	0	0	0	0
TOTALS	26	198	87	253	564	35
Total proportions	5%	35%	15%	45%		

	Saturated Calories	Mono & Poly Calories	Protein Calories	Carb Calories	Total Calories	Cholesterol (mg)

Dinner

	Saturated Calories	Mono & Poly Calories	Protein Calories	Carb Calories	Total Calories	Cholesterol (mg)
Orange-baked breast of chicken: ½ medium breast (without skin)	7	18	97	0	122	66
baked with 1 Tbsp. orange juice concentrate	0	0	3	50	53	0
1 Tbsp. safflower margarine and spices	11	91	0	0	102	0
½ cup stir-fried mixed vegetables	0	1	8	30	39	0
in 1 tsp. peanut oil	5	34	0	0	39	0
¾ cup white rice	0	1	12	149	162	0
1 tsp. safflower margarine and chicken broth	3	34	0	0	37	0
2 Tbsp. burnt onion	0	0	0	6	6	0
sautéed in scant 1 tsp. safflower margarine	2	23	0	0	25	0
3 oz. date nut cake	0	135	20	170	325	68
Noncaloric beverage	0	0	0	0	0	0
TOTALS	28	337	140	405	910	134
Total proportions	3%	37%	15%	45%		

DAY 30

Breakfast

	Saturated Calories	Mono & Poly Calories	Protein Calories	Carb Calories	Total Calories	Cholesterol (mg)
4 oz. fresh orange juice	0	0	3	52	55	0
1 oat bran English muffin	0	11	19	98	128	0
with 2 generous tsp. safflower margarine	8	66	0	0	74	3
1.5 oz. turkey sausage	20	33	37	0	90	34
Noncaloric beverage	0	0	0	0	0	0
TOTALS	28	110	59	150	347	37
Total proportions	8%	32%	17%	43%		

	Saturated Calories	Mono & Poly Calories	Protein Calories	Carb Calories	Total Calories	Cholesterol (mg)
Lunch						
2.5 oz. turkey breast sandwich	6	10	58	3	77	25
on rye roll	0	17	18	106	141	0
with ¼ large avocado	11	70	4	12	97	0
and 1 Tbsp. safflower mayo	9	88	0	2	99	0
1 apple	0	0	0	80	80	0
2 Nabisco gingersnap cookies	0	11	3	45	59	0
Noncaloric beverage	0	0	0	0	0	0
TOTALS	26	196	83	248	553	25
Total proportions	5%	35%	15%	45%		
Dinner						
3.5 oz. broiled lobster	1	4	83	5	93	71
dipped in 2½ Tbsp. safflower margarine and lemon juice	27	227	0	0	254	0
6 chilled asparagus spears	1	2	9	16	28	0
topped with 2 Tbsp. yogurt dressing	5	3	4	5	17	4
2 quick-boiled large tomato halves	0	4	5	31	40	0
topped with 1 Tbsp. grated Parmesan cheese	9	5	8	1	23	4
2 sourdough dinner rolls	0	38	18	112	168	0
1 cup orange sorbet	22	13	9	235	279	14
Noncaloric beverage	0	0	0	0	0	0
TOTALS	65	296	136	405	902	93
Total proportions	7%	33%	15%	45%		

SYNDROME X SNACKS

100 Calorie Snack	Saturated Calories	Mono & Poly Calories	Protein Calories	Carb Calories	Total Calories	Cholesterol (mg)
4 saltine crackers	0	10	5	35	50	0
Scant ½ Tbsp. peanut butter mixed with ¼ tsp. honey	5	26	9	10	50	0
TOTALS	5	36	14	45	100	0
Total proportions	5%	36%	14%	45%		
3 oz. orange juice	0	1	2	39	42	0
6 raw almonds with skins	3	31	5	6	45	0
½ slice turkey brushed lightly with vinaigrette, rolled	0	5	9	0	14	4
TOTALS	3	37	16	45	101	4
Total proportions	3%	37%	15%	45%		

Note: Each menu yields 1 serving.

100 Calorie Snack	Saturated Calories	Mono & Poly Calories	Protein Calories	Carb Calories	Total Calories	Cholesterol (mg)
2 cups air-popped popcorn, salted	0	5	6	36	47	0
½ Tbsp. peanut butter on	6	30	10	5	51	0
1 celery stalk	0	0	0	6	6	0
TOTALS	6	35	16	47	104	0
Total proportions	5%	35%	15%	45%		
¼ large apple with skin	0	1	1	19	21	0
½ slice sourdough toast	0	5	6	22	33	0
with 1½ tsp. peanut butter	5	30	8	4	47	0
TOTALS	5	36	15	45	101	0
Total proportions	5%	35%	15%	45%		

200 Calorie Snack	Saturated Calories	Mono & Poly Calories	Protein Calories	Carb Calories	Total Calories	Cholesterol (mg)
2 slices whole wheat bread or toast	0	17	18	88	123	0
1 Tbsp. peanut butter	10	58	17	9	94	0
TOTALS	10	75	35	97	217	0
Total proportions	5%	35%	16%	44%		
3 oz. low-fat yogurt	0	17	16	82	115	0
1 slice turkey	0	3	17	0	20	7
rolled in 2½ tsp. vinaigrette	0	60	0	1	61	0
TOTALS	0	80	33	83	196	7
Total proportions	0%	40%	17%	43%		
2 graham crackers (4 squares)	0	26	7	87	120	0
with 1¼ tsp. safflower margarine	5	39	0	0	44	0
¾ oz. white-meat chicken without skin	2	6	25	0	33	7
TOTALS	7	71	32	87	197	7
Total proportions	4%	36%	16%	44%		

200 Calorie Snack	Saturated Calories	Mono & Poly Calories	Protein Calories	Carb Calories	Total Calories	Cholesterol (mg)
½ large apple with skin	0	2	2	38	42	0
1 slice sourdough toast	0	10	12	44	66	0
with 1 Tbsp. peanut butter	10	60	16	8	94	0
TOTALS	10	72	30	90	202	0
Total proportions	5%	35%	15%	45%		

300 Calorie Snack						
½ large baked potato	0	1	13	134	148	0
with 1½ slices diced Canadian bacon	9	18	34	2	63	20
and 1 scant Tbsp. safflower margarine	9	84	0	0	93	0
TOTALS	18	103	47	136	304	20
Total proportions	6%	34%	15%	45%		
½ cup hummus with extra ½ tsp. safflower oil	15	95	24	100	234	0
Celery and carrot sticks	0	0	3	35	38	0
1 slice lean ham	3	7	20	0	30	11
TOTALS	18	102	47	135	302	11
Total proportions	6%	34%	15%	45%		
Guacamole: ¼ avocado	9	56	4	12	81	0
mixed with ⅓ cup low-fat cottage cheese and seasonings	3	1	34	7	45	4
¾ oz. tortilla chips	0	52	7	56	115	0
¼ cup sorbet	0	0	1	60	61	0
TOTALS	12	109	46	135	302	4
Total proportions	4%	36%	15%	45%		
¾ oz. dry-roasted lite peanuts	6	33	18	15	72	0
5 cups air-popped popcorn	0	14	14	95	123	0
with 2 scant tsp. safflower margarine	6	51	0	0	57	0

300 Calorie Snack	Saturated Calories	Mono & Poly Calories	Protein Calories	Carb Calories	Total Calories	Cholesterol (mg)
4 oz. buttermilk or low-fat milk	6	4	15	24	49	5
TOTALS	18	102	47	134	301	5
Total proportions	6%	34%	15%	45%		

BIBLIOGRAPHY

Here's a chronological listing of the key papers describing the development of Syndrome X and its current status.

Albrink, M. J., and Man, E. B. (1959) Serum triglycerides in coronary artery disease. *Arch. Intern. Med.* 103:4–8.

Yalow, R. S., and Berson, S. A. (1960) Immunoassay of endogenous plasma insulin in man. *J. Clin. Invest.* 39:1157–1175.

Ahrens, E. H. Jr., Hirsch, J., Oette, K., Farquhar, J. W., and Stein, Y. (1961) Carbohydrate-induced and fat-induced lipemia. *Trans. Assoc. Am. Phys.* 74:134.

Reaven, G., Calciano, A., Cody, R., Lucas, C., and Miller, R. (1963) Carbohydrate intolerance and hyperlipemia in patients with myocardial infarction without known diabetes mellitus. *J. Clin. Endocrinol. Metab.* 23:1013–1023.

Farquhar, J., Gross, R., Wagner, R., and Reaven, G. (1965) Validation of an incompletely coupled, two-compartment, non-recycling catenary model for turnover of hepatic and plasma triglyceride in man. *J. Lipid Res.* 6:119–134.

Reaven, G. M., Hill, D. B., Gross, R. C., and Farquhar, J. W. (1965) Kinetics of triglyceride turnover of very low density lipoproteins of human plasma. *J. Clin. Invest.* 44:1826–1833.

Farquhar, J. W., Frank, A., Gross, R. C., and Reaven, G. M. (1966) Glucose, insulin and triglyceride responses to high and low carbohydrate diets in man. *J. Clin. Invest.* 45:1648–1656.

Reaven, G. M., Lerner, R. L., Stern, M. P., and Farquhar, J. W. (1967) Role of insulin in endogenous hypertriglyceridemia. *J. Clin. Invest.* 46:1756–1767.

Shen, S.-W., Reaven, G. M., and Farquhar, J. W. (1970) Comparison of impedance to insulin-mediated glucose uptake in normal and diabetic subjects. *J. Clin. Invest.* 49:2151–2160.

Olefsky, J., Farquhar, J. W., and Reaven, G. M. (1973) Relationship between fasting plasma insulin level and resistance to insulin-mediated glucose uptake in normal and diabetic subjects. *Diabetes* 22:507–513.

Olefsky, J. M., Reaven, G. M., and Farquhar, J. W. (1974) Effects of weight reduction on obesity: studies of carbohydrate and lipid metabolism. *J. Clin. Invest.* 53:64–76.

Reaven, G. M., and Olefsky, J. M. (1974) Increased plasma glucose and insulin responses to high carbohydrate feedings in normal subjects. *J. Clin. Endocrinol. Metab.* 38:151–154.

Ginsberg, H., Olefsky, J., Farquhar, J. W., and Reaven, G. M. (1974) Moderate ethanol ingestion and plasma triglyceride levels. *Ann. Int. Med.* 80:143–149.

Ginsberg, H., Olefsky, J. M., and Reaven, G. M. (1974) Further evidence that insulin resistance exists in patients with chemical diabetes. *Diabetes* 23:674–678.

Miller, G. J., and Miller, N. E. (1975) Plasma-high-density-lipoprotein concentration and development of ischaemic heart-disease. *Lancet* 1:16–19.

Ginsberg, H., Olefsky, J. M., Kimmerling, G., Crapo, P., and Reaven, G. M. (1976) Induction of hypertriglyceridemia by a low-fat diet. *J. Clin. Endocrinol. Metab.* 42:729–735.

Reaven, G. M. (1979) Effect of differences in amount and kind of dietary carbohydrate on plasma glucose and insulin responses in man. *Am. J. Clin. Nutr.* 32:2568–2578.

Coulston, A., Greenfield, M., Kraemer, F., Tobey, T., and Reaven, G. M. (1980) Effect of source of dietary carbohydrate on plasma glucose and insulin responses to test meals in normal subjects. *Am. J. Clin. Nutr.* 33:1279–1282.

Tobey, T. A., Greenfield, M. S., Kraemer, F. B., and Reaven, G. M. (1981) Relationship between insulin resistance, insulin secretion, very low density lipoprotein kinetics and plasma triglyceride levels in normotriglyceridemia in man. *Metabolism* 30:165–171.

Coulston, A. M., Liu, G. C., Reaven, G. M. (1983) Plasma glucose, insulin and lipid responses to high-carbohydrate low-fat diets in normal humans. *Metabolism* 32:52–56.

Rosenthal, M., Haskell, W. L., Solomon, R., Widstrom, A., and Reaven, G. M. (1983) Demonstration of a relationship between level of physical training and insulin-stimulated glucose utilization in normal humans. *Diabetes* 32:408–411.

Liu, G. C., Coulston, A. M., and Reaven, G. M. (1983) Effect of high-carbohydrate–low-fat diets on plasma glucose, insulin and lipid responses in hypertriglyceridemic humans. *Metabolism* 32:750–753.

Hollenbeck, C. B., Chen, N., Chen, Y.-D. I., and Reaven, G. M. (1984) Relationship between the plasma insulin response to oral glucose and insulin-stimulated glucose utilization in normal subjects. *Diabetes* 33:460–463.

Liu, G., Coulston, A., Hollenbeck, C., and Reaven, G. M. (1984) The effect of sucrose content in high and low carbohydrate diets on plasma glucose, insulin, and lipid responses in hypertriglyceridemic humans. *J. Clin. Endocrinol. Metab.* 59:636–642.

Hollenbeck, C. B., Coulston, A. M., Donner, C. C., Williams, R. A., and Reaven, G. M. (1985) The effects of variations in percent of naturally occurring complex and simple carbohydrates on plasma glucose and insulin response in individuals with noninsulin-dependent diabetes mellitus. *Diabetes* 34:151–155.

Bogardus, C., Lillioja, S., Mott, D. M., Hollenbeck, C., and Reaven, G. M.

(1985) Relationship between degree of obesity and in vivo insulin action in man. *Am. J. Physiol.* 248 *(Endocrinol. Metab.* 11):E286–E291.

Hollenbeck, C. B., Haskell, W., Rosenthal, M., and Reaven, G. M. (1985) Effect of habitual physical activity on regulation of insulin-stimulated glucose disposal in older males. *J. Am. Geriatr. Soc.* 33:273–277.

Lucas, C. P., Estigarribia, J. A., Darga, L. L., and Reaven, G. M. (1985) Insulin and blood pressure in obesity. *Hypertension* 7:702–706.

Wilson, D. E., Chan, I.-F., Buchi, K. N., and Horton, S. C. (1985) Postchallenge plasma lipoprotein retinoids: chylomicron remnants in endogenous hypertriglyceridemia. *Metabolism* 34:551–558.

Castelli, W. P., Garrison, R. J., Wilson, P. W. F., Abbot, R. O., Kalonsdian, S., and Kannel, W. B. (1986) Incidence of coronary heart disease and lipoprotein cholesterol levels: the Framingham Study. *JAMA* 256:2835–2837.

Golay, A., Swislocki, A. L. M., Chen, Y.-D. I., Jaspan, J. B., and Reaven, G. M. (1986) Effect of obesity on ambient plasma glucose-free fatty acid, insulin, growth hormone, and glucagon concentrations. *J. Clin. Endocrinol. Metab.* 63:481–484.

Hollenbeck, C., and Reaven, G. M. (1987) Variations in insulin-stimulated glucose uptake in healthy individuals with normal glucose tolerance. *J. Clin. Endocrinol. Metab.* 64:1169–1173.

Fuh, M. M.-T., Shieh, S.-M., Wu, D.-A., Chen, Y.-D. I., and Reaven, G. M. (1987) Abnormalities of carbohydrate and lipid metabolism in patients with hypertension. *Arch. Int. Med.* 147:1035–1038.

Zavaroni, I., Dall'Aglio, E., Bonora, E., Alpi, O., Passeri, M., and Reaven, G. M. (1987) Evidence that multiple risk factors for coronary artery disease exist in persons with abnormal glucose tolerance. *Am. J. Med.* 83:609–612.

Rodnick, K. J., Haskell, W. L., Swislocki, A. L. M., Foley, J. E., and Reaven, G. M. (1987) Improved insulin action in muscle, liver, and adipose tissue in physically trained human subjects. *Am. J. Physiol.* 253:E489–495.

Austin, M. A., Breslow, J. L., Hennekens, C. H., Buring, J. E., Willett, W. S., and Krauss, R. M. (1988) Low-density lipoprotein subclass patterns and risk of myocardial infarction. *JAMA* 260:1917–1921.

Shen, D.-C., Shieh, S.-M., Fuh, M.-T., Wu, D.-A., Chen, Y.-D. I., and Reaven, G. M. (1988) Resistance to insulin-stimulated glucose uptake in patients with hypertension. *J. Clin. Endocrinol. Metab.* 66:580–583.

Parillo, M., Coulston, A., Hollenbeck, C., and Reaven, G. M. (1988) Effect of a low-fat diet on carbohydrate metabolism in patients with hypertension. *Hypertension* 11:244–248.

Hollenbeck, C. B., Coulston, A. M., and Reaven, G. M. (1988) Comparison of plasma glucose and insulin responses to mixed meals of high-, intermediate-, and low-glycemic potential. *Diabetes Care* 11:323–329.

Reaven, G. M. (1988) Role of insulin resistance in human disease. *Diabetes* 37:1595–1607.

Swislocki, A. L. M., Hoffman, B. B., and Reaven, G. M. (1989) Insulin resistance, glucose intolerance and hyperinsulinemia in patients with hypertension. *Am. J. Hypertens.* 2:419–423.

Zavaroni, I., Bonati, P. A., Luchetti, L., Bonora, E., Buonanno, G., Bergonzani, M., Pagliara, M., Gnudi, L., Butturini, L., Passeri, M., and Reaven, G. M. (1989) Habitual leisure-time physical activity is associated with differences in various risk factors for coronary artery disease. *J. Int. Med.* 226:417–421.

Juhan-Vague, I., Alessel, M. C., and Vague, P. (1991) Increased plasma plasminogen activator inhibitor 1 levels: a possible link between insulin resistance and atherothrombosis. *Diabetologia* 34:457–462.

Laws, A., and Reaven, G. M. (1992) Evidence for an independent relationship between insulin resistance and fasting plasma HDL-cholesterol, triglyceride and insulin concentrations. *J. Int. Med.* 231:25–30.

Facchini, F. S., Hollenbeck, C. B., Jeppesen, J., Chen Y.-D. I., and Reaven, G. M. (1992) Insulin resistance and cigarette smoking. *Lancet* 339:1128–1130.

Zavaroni, I., Mazza, S., Dall'Aglio, E., Gasparini, P., Passeri, M., and Reaven, G. M. (1992) Prevalence of hyperinsulinaemia in patients with high blood pressure. *J. Int. Med.* 231:235–240.

Sheu, W. H.-H., Jeng, C.-Y., Shieh, S.-M., Fuh, M. M.-T., Shen, D. D.-C., Chen, Y.-D. I., and Reaven, G. M. (1992) Insulin resistance and abnormal electrocardiograms in patients with high blood pressure. *Am. J. Hypertens.* 5:444–448.

Sheu, W. H.-H., Shieh, S.-M., Fuh, M. M.-T., Shen, D. D.-C., Jeng, C.-Y., Chen, Y.-D. I., and Reaven, G. M. (1993) Insulin resistance, glucose intolerance, and hyperinsulinemia. Hypertriglyceridemia versus hypercholesterolemia. *Arterio. and Thromb.* 13:367–370.

Reaven, G. M., Chen, Y.-D. I., Jeppesen, J., Maheux, P., and Krauss, R. M. (1993) Insulin resistance and hyperinsulinemia in individuals with small, dense, low-density lipoprotein particles. *J. Clin. Invest.* 92:141–146.

Young, M. H., Jeng, C.-Y., Sheu, W. H.-H., Shieh, S.-M., Fuh, M. M.-T., Chen, Y.-D. I., and Reaven, G. M. (1993) Insulin resistance, glucose intolerance, hyperinsulinemia and dyslipidemia in patients with angiographically demonstrated coronary artery disease. *Amer. J. Cardiol.* 72:458–460

Facchini, F., Chen, Y.-D. I., and Reaven, G. M. (1994) Light-to-moderate alcohol intake is associated with enhanced insulin sensitivity. *Diabetes Care* 17:115–119.

Zavaroni, I., Bonini, L., Fantuzzi, M., Dall'Aglio, E., Passeri, M., and Reaven, G. M. (1994) Hyperinsulinaemia, obesity, and Syndrome X. *J. Int. Med.* 235:51–56.

Zavaroni, I., Bonini, L., Gasparini, P., Dall'Aglio, E., Passeri, M., and Reaven, G. M. (1994) Cigarette smokers are relatively glucose intolerant, hyperinsulinemic and dyslipidemic. *Am. J. Cardiol.* 73:904–905.

Jeppesen, J., Hollenbeck, C. B., Zhou, M.-Y., Coulston, A. M., Jones, C., Chen, Y.-D. I., and Reaven, G. M. (1995) Relation between insulin resistance, hyperinsulinemia, postheparin plasma lipoprotein lipase activity, and postprandial lipemia. *Arterioscler. Thromb. Vasc. Biol.* 15:320–324.

Su, H.-Y., Sheu, W. H.-H., Chin, H.-M. L., Jeng, C.-Y., Chen, Y.-D. I., and Reaven, G. M. (1995) Effect of weight loss on blood pressure and insulin resistance in normotensive and hypertensive obese individuals. *Am. J. Hypertens.* 8:1067–1071.

Jeppesen, J., Chen, Y.-D. I., Zhou, M.-Y., Wang, T., and Reaven, G. M. (1995) Effect of variations in oral fat and carbohydrate load on postprandial lipemia. *Am. J. Clin. Nutr.* 62:1201–1205.

Golay, A., Allaz, A-F., Morel, Y., de Tonnac, N., Tankova, S., and Reaven, G. M. (1996) Similar weight loss with low- or high-carbohydrate diets. *Am J. Clin. Nutr.* 63:174–178.

Facchini, F. S., Riccardo, A., Stoohs, A., and Reaven, G. M. (1996) Enhanced sympathetic nervous system activity—the linchpin between insulin resistance, hyperinsulinemia, and heart rate. *Am. J. Hypertens.* 9:1013–1017.

Jeppesen, J., Schaaf, P., Jones, C., Zhou, M.-Y., Chen Y.-D. I., and Reaven, G. M. (1997) Effects of low-fat, high-carbohydrate diets on risk factors for ischemic heart disease in postmenopausal women. *Am. J. Clin. Nutr.* 65:1027–1033.

Carantoni, M., Abbasi, F., Warmerdam, F., Klebanov, M., Wang, P.-W., Chen, Y.-D. I., Azhar, S., and Reaven, G. M. (1998) Relationship between insulin resistance and partially oxidized LDL particles in healthy, nondiabetic volunteers. *Arterioscler. Thromb. Vasc. Biol.* 18:762–767.

Jeppesen, J., Facchini, F. S., and Reaven, G. M. (1998) Individuals with high total cholesterol/HDL cholesterol ratios are insulin resistant. *J. Int. Med.* 243:293–298.

Yip, J., Facchini, F. S., and Reaven, G. M. (1998) Resistance to insulin-mediated glucose disposal as a predictor of cardiovascular disease. *J. Clin. Endocrinol. Metab* 83:2773–2776.

Zavaroni, I., Zuccarelli, A., Gasparini, P., Massironi, P., Barilli, A., and Reaven, G. M. (1998) Can weight gain in healthy, nonobese volunteers be predicted by differences in baseline plasma insulin concentration? *J. Clin. Endocrinol. Metab.* 83:3498–3500.

McLaughlin, T., Abbasi, F., Carantoni, M., Schaaf, P., and Reaven, G. M. (1999) Differences in insulin resistance do not predict weight loss in response to hypocaloric diets in healthy obese women. *J. Clin. Endocrinol. Metab.* 84:578–581.

INDEX

ABOUT THE AUTHORS

Gerald Reaven, M.D., Professor Emeritus (Active) of Medicine at Stanford University, initiated the series of studies leading to the discovery of Syndrome X. A world-renowned endocrinologist, he has served as Director of the Division of Endocrinology and Metabolism, the Division of Gerontology, and the combined Divisions of Endocrinology-Metabolism-Gerontology, among other posts, at Stanford's School of Medicine. Dr. Reaven has received a wide array of scientific awards and is the author of over five hundred scholarly papers in *The Journal of the American Medical Association*, *The New England Journal of Medicine*, *The Lancet*, and elsewhere. He has also served as Editor in Chief of the journal *Hormone and Metabolic Research*. He lives in Stanford, California.

Terry Kristen Strom, M.B.A., former Chief Business Officer of the General Clinical Research Center and Business Director of Pediatrics at Stanford University, has authored dozens of articles on health care administration and management for the *Journal of the Association of Administrators in Academic Pediatrics* and various other health care publications. She lives in Palo Alto, California.

Barry Fox, Ph.D., is the bestselling coauthor of *The Arthritis Cure* and many other books. He lives in Los Angeles.

Syn X Bar

Chocolate Chunk Almond Brownie

$5.00 Off Plus Free Shipping on One Box of 12 SYN X BARS

The Syn X Bar provides energy in a form that complements the Syndrome X Diet, formulated to boost your defenses against the multiple disease manifestations of Syndrome X and to promote good overall health. This bar is a product of more than 35 years of clinical research of specific dietary strategies shown to improve cardiovascular wellness by helping you achieve healthy blood sugar, insulin, cholesterol and triglyceride (blood fat) levels. The Syn X Bar conforms to Dr Reaven's Syndrome X Diet of 15% protein, 40% fat (mostly monounsaturated), and 45% carbohydrate. When the Syn X Bar is used in conjunction with the Syndrome X Diet it can help those who are insulin resistant reduce their risk of heart attack and other manifestations of Syndrome X. For more information and free use of the Nutrition Analysis Tool to monitor your diet, visit the website www.syndromeXweb.com.

To order Syn X Bars call 1-877-915-4045 or send a check for $14.95 payable to Shaman Pharmaceuticals, Inc. with the coupon below to:

> Shaman Pharmaceuticals, Inc.
> Syn X Bar Box Discount-Bk
> 213 East Grand Avenue
> South San Francisco, CA 94080-4812

Enclosed is my check for $14.95. Please send me a box of Syn X Bars to:

Your Name_____

Street Address _____

City _____ State _____

Zip code_____

Email address (Optional) _____